For Elsevier:

Commissioning Editor: Robert Edwards
Development Editor: Rebecca Gleave
Project Manager: Jess Thompson
Design Direction: George Ajayi

eye essentials

cataract

Raman Malhotra FRCOphth
Consultant Ophthalmic Surgeon, Queen Victoria Hospital, East Grinstead, UK

SERIES EDITORS
Sandip Doshi PhD MCOptom
Optometrist in private practice, Hove, East Sussex, UK
Examiner, College of Optometrists, London, UK
Formerly Clinical Editor, Optician

William Harvey MCOptom
Visiting Clinician and Director of Visual Impairment Clinic, City University, London, UK
Professional Programme Tutor for Boots Opticians Ltd
Clinical Editor, Optician, Reed Business Information, Sutton, UK

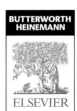

BUTTERWORTH
HEINEMANN

ELSEVIER

EDINBURGH LONDON NEW YORK OXFORD
PHILADELPHIA ST LOUIS SYDNEY TORONTO 2008

BUTTERWORTH
HEINEMANN
ELSEVIER

© 2008, Elsevier Limited. All rights reserved.
First published 2008

ISBN 978-0-08-044977-7

British Library Cataloguing in Publication Data
A catalogue record for this book is available from the British Library

Library of Congress Cataloging in Publication Data
A catalog record for this book is available from the Library of Congress

Working together to grow
libraries in developing countries

www.elsevier.com | www.bookaid.org | www.sabre.org

ELSEVIER   BOOK AID International   Sabre Foundation

ELSEVIER   your source for books, journals and multimedia in the health sciences

www.elsevierhealth.com

The publisher's policy is to use paper manufactured from sustainable forests

Printed in China

Contents

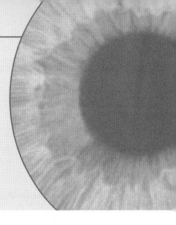

Contents

Contributors

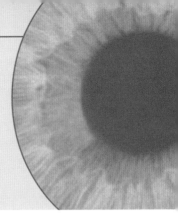

Sally J Embleton MCOptom PhD
Optometrist, UK

Kenneth CS Fong MA MB BChir FRCOphth
Specialist Registrar in Ophthalmology, Moorfields Eye Hospital,
London, UK

Samer Hamada MD MSc MRCOphth FRCSEd
Clinical Fellow in Paediatric Ophthalmology, Great Ormond Street
Hospital for Children, London, UK
Formerly, Clinical Fellow in Cornea and Refractive Surgery,
Corneoplastic Unit, Queen Victoria Hospital, East Grinstead, UK

Raman Malhotra FRCOphth
Consultant Ophthalmic and Oculoplastic Surgeon
Corneoplastic Unit, Queen Victoria Hospital, East Grinstead, UK

Richard Packard MD DO FRCS FRCOphth
Consultant Ophthalmic Surgeon
Director, Arnott Eye Associates, London, UK
Clinical Director, Prince Charles Eye Unit, King Edward VII
Hospital, Windsor, UK

Manoj V Parulekar MS FRCSEd
Consultant Ophthalmologist, Birmingham Children's Hospital,
Birmingham, UK

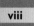

CK Patel BSc FRCOphth
Consultant Ophthalmic Surgeon, Oxford Eye Hospital, Radcliffe
Infirmary, Oxford, UK

Helen Pointer RN OND
Senior Matron, Corneoplastic Unit,
Queen Victoria Hospital, East Grinstead, UK

Foreword by the series editors

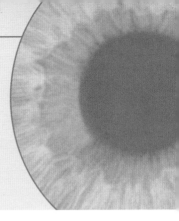

Eye Essentials is a series of books intended to cover the core skills required by the eye care practitioner in general and/or specialized practice. It consists of books covering a wide range of topics, ranging from: routine eye examination to assessment and management of low vision; assessment and investigative techniques to digital imaging; case reports and law to contact lenses.

Authors known for their interest and expertise in their particular subject have contributed books to this series. The reader will know many of them, as they have published widely within their respective fields. Each author has addressed key topics in their subject in a practical rather than theoretical approach, hence each book has a particular relevance to everyday practice.

Each book in the series follows a similar format and has been designed to enable the reader to ascertain information easily and quickly. Each chapter has been produced in a user-friendly format, thus providing the reader with a rapid-reference book that is easy to use in the consulting room or in the practitioner's free time.

Optometry and dispensing optics are continually developing professions, with the emphasis in each being redefined as we learn more from research and as technology stamps its mark. The *Eye Essentials* series is particularly relevant to the practitioner's requirements and as such will appeal to students, graduates sitting professional examinations and qualified practitioners alike. We hope you enjoy reading these books as much as we have enjoyed producing them.

Sandip Doshi
Bill Harvey

Foreword

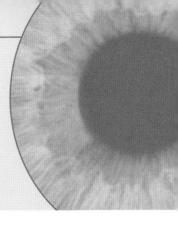

Patient care pathways, optometric direct referral, improved efficiency, reduction in waiting times, cost containment and shared care – just some of the buzzwords being used at the moment in the ever changing world of eyecare provision in the United Kingdom. Ultimately, efficiency and cost containment are among the main drivers, however there is no doubt that the roles of professionals will evolve, change and expand to encompass knowledge well outside previously conceived boundaries. This is where this book – *Cataract*, a component of the *Eye Essentials* series – fits right in and fills a gap in available resources for the optometrist involved in cataract care.

This book provides a comprehensive overview of cataract and its surgical correction in 2007. Like any subject, thorough knowledge is only gained from first understanding the fundamentals. The contents of the book have been carefully thought out and the authors have made a deliberate effort to remain concise. Thus every chapter makes important reading for the optometrist involved in care of the cataract patient, whether it be direct involvement in shared care or in the long-term care of the pseudophakic patient.

Cataract surgery is the most common surgical procedure performed and with the "baby boomers" now well into their sixth decade the numbers of procedures are set to increase. Demands of patients are also increasing and fortunately we live in very good times for eye surgery and so are well able to cater to this demand. Cataract surgeries are now being performed earlier, as soon as visual quality becomes significant and affects the ability of the individual to function. Cataract surgery has also become more and more of a refractive procedure and ophthalmologists now have the ability to make emmetropia their goal. Indeed, this is now the expectation and no matter what level of previous refractive error, and level of astigmatism, there now exists a means of attaining full correction. Available lenses and adjunct procedures are addressed in some detail in this book. Presbyopia is the next frontier and considerable advance has been made already, with more coming in the pipeline. Attention to detail and thorough patient counselling are vital to success in adding presbyopic correction, and again I envisage an increasingly important role for the optometrist in this area. The management of patients' expectations through a good understanding of what is available is undoubtedly a shared-care function.

No surgical procedure is without problem and complication and the same applies to cataract surgery. Beware the surgeon who indicates they have no complications, they are either being untruthful or not doing any surgery! Fortunately, serious complications are rare, however the most severe need early identification and rectification to avoid ocular morbidity. This is well addressed in this book and will probably be the most referenced area. Nevertheless, the text cannot totally replace direct experience and the cataract optometrist will benefit by spending time at a local cataract unit on a periodic basis.

Raman Malhotra and his well-known contributors are to be congratulated on this comprehensive and well-written text.

Sheraz M Daya MD FACP FACS FRCSEd FRCOphth
Director and Consultant
Corneoplastic Unit and Eye Bank
Queen Victoria Hospital NHS Foundation Trust
East Grinstead, UK

Acknowledgements

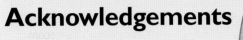

I would like to sincerely thank all my co-authors for agreeing to contribute to this project with their expertise and valuable spare time and for patiently putting up with my numerous emails and extra requests along the way. I would also especially like to thank Kavita, Gaurav and Shyam, from whom my time was taken.

Raman Malhotra

1

The ageing lens and classification of cataracts

Kenneth CS Fong

Introduction

The primary functions of the crystalline lens are to transmit incident light and to focus it on the retina. This requires that the lens is transparent, a condition dependent on the highly regular organization of the cells of the lens and the high degree of order of the proteins in the lens cytoplasm. The protein concentration in lens fibre cells is extremely high, resulting in an index of refraction significantly greater than that of the surrounding fluids, and so enabling the lens to refract incident light. Cataract occurs when the lens loses its transparency by either scattering or absorbing light such that visual acuity is compromised.

Cataracts can result from genetic, metabolic, nutritional or environmental insults, or they may be secondary to other ocular or systemic diseases such as diabetes or retinal degenerative diseases (see box). By far the most important risk factor is age; ageing-related cataract constitutes the great majority of all cataracts and is a major public health problem worldwide. In developing countries, where the availability of surgical facilities is limited, ageing-related cataract is the leading cause of blindness. Because at present there is no efficacious non-surgical therapy for cataract, the problem is expected to increase in magnitude in

---

Causes of cataracts

- Ageing
- Inheritance
- Metabolic disorders, e.g. Lowe's syndrome, hypocalcaemia
- Diabetes
- Toxicity, e.g. drug-induced (steroids, amiodarone), chemical, metal ions
- Nutrition
- Physical dehydration
- Trauma
- Radiation
- Eye disease, e.g. glaucoma, uveitis, post-vitrectomy
- Systemic disease, e.g. atopy, renal failure

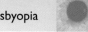

coming decades as the world population becomes progressively older.

Lens growth

Although the lens grows throughout life, none of the cells are cast off. Component cells are added to the lens as time goes by, with those in the centre being as old as the individual. The lens grows by regular addition of fibres to the lens mass. Growth rate is not uniform throughout the human lifespan, and it appears to be maximal in foetal life. Foetal lens mass increases by about 180 mg/year (lens mass is 90 mg at birth), but the growth rate drops significantly after birth and is 1.3 mg/year between 10 and 90 years of age. Estimates of average lens density suggest that protein content remains relatively constant at around 33% of the wet weight over the age span.

The dimensions of the lens change in a complex manner as the lens grows. In early foetal life, the lens is almost perfectly spherical, but by birth the sagittal profile is ellipsoidal as equatorial growth outstrips growth in the sagittal plane. At birth, equatorial lens diameter is about 6.5 mm while sagittal width is about 3 mm. By the age of 90 years, this changes to about 10 mm in the equatorial plane and 6 mm in the sagittal plane.

Presbyopia

Loss of accommodative power is a lens-related problem initiated in infancy. This steady loss of accommodation is completed by about the age of 50 years and is coupled with difficulty in restoring focus from near to far. The factors responsible for presbyopia are multiple and their relative contributions to the presbyopic state are not established.

Some of the factors involved are:

- forward shift of the apical part of the ciliary body with age, which reduces the function of the muscle

- increase in the connective tissue of the ciliary muscle
- increased stiffness of the cortex and nucleus of the lens
- increased curvature of the anterior lens surface, which reduces the ability of ciliary muscle contraction to change the lens shape during accommodation.

Oxidation and lens ageing

Oxidative damage to lens constituents, including nucleic acids, proteins and lipids, is believed to be a primary factor in ageing-related cataract. That oxidative stress can be cataractogenic is clear from abundant data demonstrating, both in animals and in humans, that exposure of the eye to X-rays or to high levels of other types of radiation, including ultraviolet (UV) and microwave, can cause cataract, with definitive oxidative effects in the lens. Likewise, exposure to hyperbaric oxygen, either experimentally in animals or therapeutically in patients, can cause cataracts. Further support for the oxidation hypothesis comes from epidemiological studies that have found an association between increased exposure to sunlight, particularly its UV component, and ageing-related cataract.

Scatter and absorption changes

The young human lens is colourless and transmits almost 100% of the incident light. With age, both scatter and absorption of optical radiation increase, with the result that the lens becomes yellow.

The absorption of optical radiation by the lens increases exponentially with age. The rise in absorption is greatest for wavelengths at the blue end of the spectrum (460 nm), which is due to accumulation of yellow chromophores. Increasing yellowing of the lens and absorption of wavelengths at the blue end of the spectrum plays a protective role against the harmful effects of optical radiation on the macula. This is one of the factors that led to the development of yellow-tinted intraocular lenses for cataract surgery, e.g. Acrysof Natural (Alcon).

Classification of cataracts

There appears to be three major types of ageing-related cataracts—cortical, nuclear and posterior subcapsular—which differ both in the location in which the opacity initially appears and in the pathology underlying the opacification. Many risk factors may be common to all three types of ageing-related cataracts, and although cataracts often begin as a pure type, as they mature they typically become mixed cataracts. The main types of cataracts seen in clinical practice are summarized in the box below.

Objective classification schemes (see box) use photographic standards to subdivide each major type into grades. These grades are based on density and colour (in the case of the nucleus) or according to the anatomical area of the cataract (in the case of the cortical and posterior subcapsular areas). One may directly compare a patient's lens as seen on the slit lamp with a photographic copy of the various standard grades, as set up in the various classification schemes (clinical grading), or one may take photographs of the lens being studied and later grade the photographs according to the classification scheme used (photographic grading).

Types of cataracts

- Cortical
- Nuclear
- Posterior subcapsular
- Mixed
- Mature and hypermature
- Capsular
- Anterior subcapsular
- Retrodots
- Congenital and juvenile—total or partial
- Traumatic

> ## Objective classification schemes for cataracts
>
> - Lens Opacities Classification System II and III (LOCS II and LOCS III)
> - Oxford Cataract Classification System
> - Beaver Dam Eye Study
> - Age Related Eye Diseases Study (AREDS)

Cortical cataracts

Cortical cataracts (Figure 1.1) are the most common of the three major pure cataract types. It is notable that although certain types of cataracts may initially occur as pure types, as a cataract progresses it eventually becomes mixed as the other anatomical areas become affected. The cortical layer is less compact than the nucleus and is therefore more prone to becoming overhydrated as a result of electrolyte imbalance, which eventually leads to disruption of the lens cortical fibres, as demonstrated in diabetes and galactosaemia. It has therefore been proposed that this type of cataract may be partly caused by osmotic stress. Early changes may include signs such as vacuoles, water clefts and lamellar separation. These changes may come and go over time, but eventually they may predispose the patient to damage and irreversible opacification of some fibres.

Most cortical cataracts remain in the periphery for many years, even decades, before the central axis of the lens becomes involved, causing loss of vision late in the development of the cataract. Patients with this type of cataract are usually reassured

Figure 1.1   Cortical cataract

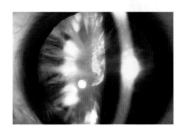

that their cataracts may not decrease their vision for a good number of years and that they do not need to worry about undergoing cataract surgery until it happens.

It has been observed that patients may have an advanced grade of cortical cataract (e.g. cortical opacities covering the entire anterior cortical and posterior cortical areas) and yet have 6/12 or better Snellen visual acuity under standard testing conditions. This occurs especially when the cortical cataract is of a low density, allowing enough light to reach the macula to stimulate it adequately; however, these patients have severe glare disability as documented by the brightness acuity tester (BAT) (Figure 1.2) such that under simulated bright lights their visual acuity may decrease to 6/24 or worse. They also have decreased contrast sensitivity. These patients tend to do well indoors but have difficulty driving during bright, sunny days and at night because of oncoming headlights. Treatment in these cases must be decided on an individual basis.

Nuclear cataracts

Nuclear cataracts (Figure 1.3) appear to be an exaggeration of the normal sclerosis or hardening and yellowing of the nucleus in

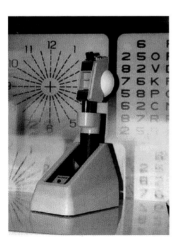

Figure 1.2 Brightness acuity tester (Mentor O&O, Inc., Norwell, MA)

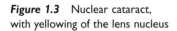

Figure 1.3 Nuclear cataract, with yellowing of the lens nucleus

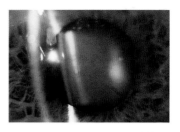

older adult patients. Studies have documented a gradual increase in optical density of the nucleus with increasing age in normal adults with 6/6 vision.

Nuclear cataracts tend to progress slowly, with the visual acuity of patients remaining in the 6/9 range for prolonged periods. The refractive index of the lens changes as the nucleus progressively hardens, usually resulting in increasing myopia and astigmatism. In some patients this is accompanied by optical distortion, especially of distant images, while near vision remains in the N6 range. This is especially true in patients with high axial myopia, in whom refraction sometimes fails to provide adequate restoration of distance vision.

This type of cataract is best seen with the narrow-beam direct illumination employed by the slit lamp, which reveals the colour and generalized haze or opalescence of the nucleus. In the early stages, the two halves (cotyledons) of the embryonic nucleus remain visible. Later, the entire nucleus appears as a homogeneous mass in contrast to the cortex. Retroillumination may show the 'oil droplet' effect. Sometimes one may notice crystals in the lens nucleus (Christmas tree cataract).

Nuclear cataracts are associated with physiochemical changes in the lens structural proteins (α-, β- and γ-crystallins). These proteins undergo oxidation, non-enzymatic glycosylation, proteolysis, deamidation, phosphorylation and carbamylation, leading to aggregation and formation of high-molecular-weight proteins. Chemical modification of the nuclear lens protein leads to yellowing, followed by browning, and in advanced stages blackening.

Posterior subcapsular cataracts

Posterior subcapsular cataracts (PSCs) (Figure 1.4) are less
frequently encountered than nuclear or cortical cataracts but
often occur in combination with them in the later stages. PSCs
are easily noticed on retroillumination as they are usually located
centrally, and they may interfere with funduscopy. In early stages,
patients usually complain of subjective symptoms such as glare
disability and difficulty focusing on objects, especially for near.
This is due to the fact that when the pupil constricts during
accommodation, the light entering the eye becomes concentrated
centrally, where the PSC is also located, causing light scattering
and interfering with the ability of the eye to focus an image on
the macula. In addition, these opacities lie at or near the nodal
point of the eye, further interfering with focusing the image on
the macula.

This type of cataract may be examined with direct illumination,
using the narrow and broad beams of the slit lamp to show the
characteristic granular inner surface immediately in front of the
posterior capsule. The problem with this technique, however, is
that patients may not tolerate any prolonged direct illumination
due to intolerable glare. Retroillumination is therefore more
useful for revealing the outline of the opacity, as it is usually seen
as an 'island' in the centre of the posterior capsule, which is
further highlighted by the shadow cast by the opacities.

In the early stages of a PSC, however, the dust-like particles
that might be noticeable in the central posterior subcapsular

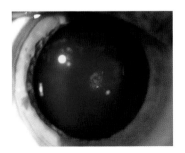

Figure 1.4 Posterior
subcapsular cataract

area with direct illumination disappear or are difficult to see with retroillumination. Eventually, this 'dusting' becomes dense enough to cast a shadow and thus to appear on retroillumination. The smooth orange background of the fundus helps to highlight the rough, irregular pseudopodia-like edges of the central opacity. In advanced stages, the PSC may become a thick, calcified plaque.

PSCs may also result from irradiation or steroid ingestion, or they may be associated with diabetes, high myopia, retinal degeneration (e.g. retinitis pigmentosa) and gyrate atrophy.

Mixed cataracts

Mixed cataracts are where more than one variety of cataract occur together. A cataract normally starts as one type, but it may eventually become a mixed cataract as the other lens regions become involved in the degenerative process. A mixed cataract indicates that the cataract has already advanced to some degree and that its progression should be watched more closely. Patients with mixed cataracts tend to have more visual symptoms.

Mature cataracts

The lens may swell and increase in volume rapidly because of rapid hydration of the lens cortex. Complete opacification of the lens is called a mature cataract (Figure 1.5). If the liquefied cortical material is not reabsorbed, the solid nucleus may 'sink' to the bottom of the lens bag (Morgagnian cataract), this is rarely seen in the UK. Reabsorption of the milky cortex causes reduction in the lens volume, causing the capsule to form folds.

Figure 1.5 Mature cataract, with folds on the anterior lens capsule

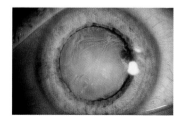

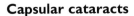

Capsular cataracts

The lens capsule may develop localized opacities in ageing-related cataracts. However, they may also occur in uveitis in association with posterior synechiae or secondary to injury caused by drugs, radiation or trauma. Localized central capsular cataracts (polar cataracts) can occur in the anterior and posterior capsule. They are usually congenital, although they may also be secondary to trauma.

Polar cataracts (Figure 1.6) are usually dense, localized and non-progressive. Because they are stable, many patients may be able to tolerate them and may retain good, adequate vision with conservative treatment (e.g. dilation of the pupil, wearing sunglasses on bright days, optical correction). For the surgeon, extra care has to be taken when removing this type of cataract as there is a high risk of posterior capsule rupture during surgery.

Anterior subcapsular cataracts

In contrast to PSCs, anterior subcapsular cataracts consist of multilayering of the anterior lens epithelium and deposition of abnormal lens capsule. They may occur together with PSCs. They may also result from local injury or irritation, as in uveitis, or injury due to chemicals or radiation.

Retrodots

Retrodots are round, translucent opacities that usually occur in the deep cortex or perinuclear region. In general they do not seem to affect vision until a mixed cataract appears (nuclear or

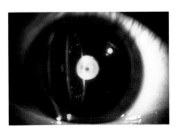

Figure 1.6 Posterior polar cataract

cortical), and patients may have retrodots for years and still retain good vision.

Congenital and juvenile cataracts

Congenital cataracts are detected at birth, whereas juvenile cataracts develop during the first 12 years of life. Both range from mild and benign to advanced and sight-threatening. Congenital cataracts are the third most common cause of blindness in children.

The following is a morphologic classification of congenital cataracts:

I. **Total or complete**
    These cataracts are completely opaque or hazy at birth. Most of these are associated with systemic disorders or abnormalities such as galactosemia, rubella, and Lowe's syndrome. They may also be hereditary (autosomal dominant or autosomal recessive).
II. **Partial or incomplete**
A. **Anterior and posterior polar cataracts** (Figure 1.6):
    These cataracts involve the lens capsule in the anterior or posterior pole of the lens. They are sometimes associated with a localized anatomical abnormality in the region. For example, posterior polar cataracts commonly occur in cases of posterior lenticonus. They may cause severe visual symptoms because they are closer to the nodal point of the eye; however, they are usually stable, and patients may do well with conservative measures. The familial type is bilateral and inherited as an autosomal-dominant trait.
B. **Zonular cataracts:** In this type of cataract only a region or zone of the lens is opaque. Zonular cataracts may be stationary, but they may also progress. There are various subtypes:
    1. Lamellar: This is the most common type of congenital cataract. Such cases are usually bilateral and symmetric, and the density of opacification may vary considerably (Figure 1.7). Less opaque lamellar cataracts may be

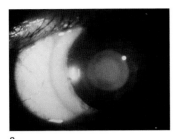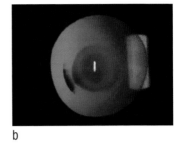

a   b

Figure 1.7 Lamellar cataract—(a) direct illumination view and
(b) retroillumination view

compatible with good vision and require minimal medical
intervention (e.g. optical correction, therapeutic mydriasis).
These cataracts may be inherited as an autosomal-
dominant trait, but in some cases they may be attributed to
a transient intrauterine toxic agent, affecting only the layer
of cells developing at the time of foetal exposure.

2. **Stellate:** These cataracts affect the region of the sutures.
They may be Y-shaped if the cataract occurs in the
intrauterine stage of development as the sutures have this
configuration during this period. Anterior sutural cataracts
are Y-shaped; posterior sutural cataracts are shaped like an
inverted Y. Sutural cataracts that develop later on have a
more stellate shape, in keeping with the shape of the
sutures after birth.

3. **Nuclear:** These cataracts are usually bilateral and involve
the foetal or embryonal nucleus. They may be inherited as
an autosomal-dominant, autosomal-recessive or X-linked
trait.

4. **Coronary:** These cataracts are radial, club-shaped discrete
opacities located in the cortex. They are called 'coronary'
because their appearance is like the top of a crown.
Because of their peripheral location they do not decrease
visual acuity. Coronary cataracts are dominantly inherited
and have been described in cases of Down's syndrome and
myotonic dystrophy.

5. Cerulean: These cataracts consist of small, discrete opacities that have a distinct bluish hue. These opacities are located in the cortex, are non-progressive and do not cause visual symptoms. They may be present together with other congenital cataracts.

C. Membranous cataracts: These cataracts are thin but dense and contain fibrous tissue. They may occur when lens proteins are reabsorbed (e.g. traumatized lens; see following section), such that the anterior and posterior lens capsules fuse, producing a dense membrane.

Traumatic cataract

Cataracts can occur secondary to trauma to the lens. The morphological characteristics differ between cataracts due to blunt trauma and cataracts secondary to penetrating trauma. Cataracts secondary to blunt trauma often have a rosette-shaped appearance or are of the PSC variety. In cataracts secondary to penetrating trauma, the size of the opening in the lens capsule determines the morphology of the cataract. When the opening is large, the whole lens is cataractous; when the opening is small, it may sometimes seal by itself and leave behind an opacity that is localized to the site of penetration.

Summary

There are many subjective ways of classifying cataracts, but the most commonly employed is by anatomical location of lens opacities, i.e. cortical, nuclear and posterior subcapsular. Several types of clinical grading and photographic standards to aid the clinician have been developed to grade each type of cataract.

Further reading

Chitkara D.K. and Colin J. (2006). Morphology and visual effects of lens opacities of cataract. In: *Ophthalmology*. Ed: Yanoff M. and Duker J.S. Elsevier, Chapter 37.

Datiles III M.B. and Magno B.V. (2005). Cataract: Clinical types. In: *Duane's Clinical Ophthalmology*. Ed: Tasman W. and Jaegar E.A. Lippincott, Williams and Wilkins, Chapter 73.

Kuszak J.R., Al-Ghoul K.J. and Costello M.J. (2005). Pathology of age-related human cataracts. In: *Duane's Clinical Ophthalmology*. Ed: Tasman W. and Jaegar E.A. Lippincott, Williams and Wilkins, Chapter 71B.

Patel C.K. and Bron A.J. (2001). The ageing lens. *Optometry Today*, May: 27–31.

Zigler Jr. J.S. and Datiles III M.B. (2005). Pathogenesis of cataracts. In: *Duane's Clinical Ophthalmology*. Ed: Tasman W. and Jaegar E.A. Lippincott, Williams and Wilkins. Chapter 72B.

2

Assessment of the patient with cataract

Kenneth CS Fong and Raman Malhotra

Introduction

Management of the patient with cataract is a multidisciplinary team affair, in which optometrists play a key role. Optometrists need to be able to take a good history from the patient to determine if cataracts are actually affecting the patient's quality of life and that treatment would be of benefit. They should also be able to explain what cataracts are and their management without causing undue alarm to the patient. The primary purpose in managing a patient with cataract is to improve functional vision and therefore the patient's quality of life.

When should a patient be referred for cataract surgery?

Cataracts are often discovered on routine optometric examination and patients are usually asymptomatic. It is imperative to discuss with the patient whether they actually want cataract surgery before referring them to an ophthalmologist. Guidelines for cataract surgery from the Royal College of Ophthalmologists suggest that patients should be referred for cataract surgery if there is sufficient cataract to account for their visual symptoms and that these limit their quality of life and ability to work or drive, irrespective of Snellen visual acuity. Cataract surgery may be appropriate for a patient with good Snellen visual acuity but who complains of glare or problems with night driving. Conversely, surgery may be inappropriate for a non-driver with adequate reading vision but poor distance acuity if they are happy with their current level of vision. Simply put, the risks of cataract surgery should be outweighed by the anticipated benefits to an individual patient's daily activities.

Once a cataract is diagnosed, the optometrist should:

1. Determine the overall effect of cataract on visual function and the well-being of the patient

These assessments will serve as the basis for a decision

whether to recommend cataract surgery. A careful inquiry should be made into the patient's daily, occupational, leisure, and social activities, and document any cataract-related impairment. If the patient holds a driving licence then the legal visual requirements for and any symptoms affecting driving should be determined.

2. **Identify coexisting ocular conditions as predictors of poor visual outcome following surgery**

   Significant coexisting conditions include the following:

   - **corneal pathology**: this includes corneal opacities, degenerative disorders, hereditary conditions (in particular, Fuch's endothelial dystrophy and corneal oedema) and ectasia
   - **glaucoma**: uncontrolled intraocular pressure or visual field loss
   - **uveitis**
   - **pseudoexfoliation**: most commonly found in the Scandinavian or northern European population. Characterized by a deposition of a white fluffy material (similar to amyloid) on the anterior lens capsule with a relatively clear zone corresponding to the movement of the iris (Figure 2.1). In addition, this material is deposited on the zonules, iris pigment epithelium, ciliary epithelium, trabecular meshwork and cornea. The pupil often fails to dilate fully, potentially making cataract surgery more challenging. This

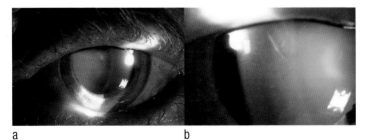

a   b

Figure 2.1 (a) Pseudoexfoliation, (b) the same eye under greater magnification showing pseudoexfoliation deposits on the anterior lens capsule

condition may lead to glaucoma, as well as to weakness of the zonules. Complications may therefore also be encountered during cataract surgery due to zonular dialysis.

- **vitreous opacification**
- **diabetic retinopathy**: cataract surgery in diabetic patients has been associated with a higher incidence of post-operative complications (also see *Diabetes and the eye* in this series), including fibrinous uveitis, posterior capsule opacification, anterior segment neovascularization, accelerated progression of diabetic retinopathy and macular oedema. Post-operative visual acuity may therefore be poor. A number of issues relating to cataract surgery in diabetes remain incompletely resolved, including appropriate timing of surgery, determinants of visual outcome, impact of surgery on retinopathy, and optimal management of postoperative macular oedema. Patients with diabetic retinopathy need to be carefully examined prior to cataract surgery.

The key question is whether the patient has proliferative diabetic retinopathy (PDR) or macular oedema. If either or both cases are present, it is essential to counsel the patient about the guarded prognosis to their vision after cataract surgery.

If the patient has PDR, this needs to be treated as much as possible with pan-retinal laser photocoagulation (PRP) prior to cataract surgery. If the cataract is severe enough to preclude a good view of the retina for adequate PRP then urgent cataract surgery is warranted. It may be then possible to perform PRP with an indirect viewing system at the time of surgery after the cataract has been removed, or if this is not possible PRP should be arranged within one week of surgery. If PDR is present, cataract surgery will accelerate its progression, and the visual results can be poor if the PDR is not treated aggressively.

Macular oedema may be difficult to detect clinically if a cataract is present. If macular oedema is seen prior to cataract surgery, this should be treated with focal or grid laser as necessary. A pre-operative fundus fluorescein angiogram is helpful in identifying areas of macular oedema and leakage from active new vessels. If macular oedema is present at the time of cataract surgery, it will most likely worsen with time if left untreated.

All patients with diabetic retinopathy who have had cataract surgery need to be seen within one week of their operation for a dilated retinal examination. Any evidence of PDR or macular oedema should be treated as soon as possible to prevent progression of the disease. Cataract surgery appears to cause progression of diabetic retinopathy but not diabetic maculopathy.

- **age-related macular degeneration** (ARMD): patients with ARMD may suffer further deterioration of their visual acuity due to cataract, and the majority would experience significant improvements in quality of life as well as in visual function following cataract surgery. This is particularly the case with increasing severity of cataract, irrespective of the degree of ARMD. Cataracts are known to cause reduced distance and near visual acuity as well as contrast sensitivity by reducing the quality and physical contrast in the retinal image. The reduced contrast sensitivity is a consequence of forward scatter of light from the lens, producing the effect of veiling glare, which obviously improves when cataracts are removed. Therefore, daily living activities that involve the detection of objects at low physical contrasts are likely to benefit from cataract surgery despite the presence of ARMD. Furthermore, peripheral retinal function, particularly that for lower spatial frequencies, may improve.

Of concern are the findings by some studies that suggest that eyes with ARMD that undergo routine cataract surgery are at a slightly greater risk of progression to wet ARMD in comparison with the fellow eye. This implies that cataract surgery may be an important possible risk factor in progression of macular degeneration. Patients with ARMD must decide whether to proceed with cataract surgery in the face of uncertain information about the ultimate result.

- **retinal vascular disorders**: signs of previous branch or central retinal vein or arterial occlusion may be subtle but they should be suspected, particularly if the loss of visual function is not commensurate with the degree of cataract.
- **no view of fundus**: lack of a clear retinal view may be due to significant corneal opacity, dense or mature cataract or a vitreous opacity. This influences the ability to assess retinal and optic nerve function. Most importantly, retinal detachment or intraocular tumour must be excluded, which may require the use of a B-scan ultrasound. Where a significant opacity precludes retinal visualization, optic nerve and retinal function may be clinically assessed by way of confrontational visual field testing and the ability to detect light in all four quadrants of the uniocular visual field. Furthermore, the response of the pupil to light and the presence of a relative afferent pupillary defect (RAPD) should be determined. Cataract, even if mature, should not cause an RAPD.
- **amblyopia**
- **optic nerve or neurological disease.**

The 'only eye' patient

Patients who only have good vision in one eye will naturally be more concerned about the prospect of surgery. Modern cataract surgery carries much lower risk than in the past, and in general the threshold for intervention should not be set at a higher level for such patients. However, increased sensitivity in counselling is required.

Urgent cataract surgery

There are unusual circumstances in which cataract surgery should be expedited. When a cataract is mature, an inflammatory reaction may occur with acutely raised intraocular pressure.

Cataract surgery is also expedited in narrow-angle glaucoma, particular if a significant phacomorphic component exists. Such patients should be referred urgently to an ophthalmologist for surgery.

Recent research has also revealed the interesting observation that in older patients, cataracts may play an important role in the causation of car accidents, falling accidents resulting in fractures, and functional decline. Hence, earlier visual rehabilitation through modern cataract surgery with intraocular lens implantation is becoming the norm rather than an option.

Visual standards for driving

The following are the minimum visual acuity standards required for driving as applied by the Driving and Vehicle Licensing Agency (DVLA). There is also a visual field standard but this is not statutory, unlike the visual acuity standards. The visual field standard for ordinary driving is currently defined as:

> a field of at least 120° on the horizontal measured using the Goldmann III4e setting or the equivalent. In addition there should be no significant defect in the binocular field which encroaches within 20° of fixation either above or below the horizontal meridian.

Group 1 drivers (car and other light vehicles)

All drivers are required by law to read a standard sized number plate in good light at 20.5 m. In September 2001 the new format number plate was introduced on all new registrations and on replacement number plates. The characters are narrower than on the previous number plate and the new format plate should be read at 20 m. The number plate test is absolute in law and not open to interpretation. A driver who is unable to satisfy this requirement is guilty of an offence under section 96 of the Road Traffic Act 1988. The number plate test corresponds to a binocular visual acuity of approximately 6/10 Snellen acuity. However, it is important to stress that visual acuity measurements in a consulting room may not correspond to the ability to read the standard number plate at the roadside.

Group 2 drivers (large goods and passenger carrying vehicles)

Since January 1st 1997 all new Group 2 applicants must by law have:

- a visual acuity of at least 6/9 in the better eye *and*
- a visual acuity of at least 6/12 in the worse eye *and*
- if these are achieved by correction, the *uncorrected* visual acuity in each eye must be no less than 3/60.

Pre-operative hospital assessment

The principal aims of the pre-operative hospital assessment are listed in the box below.

The minimum ocular examination should include testing for a relative afferent pupillary defect, confrontational visual field examination, assessment of the ocular surface to exclude blepharitis, conjunctivitis, dry eyes or obvious nasolacrimal blockage. During the slit lamp examination, special attention should be paid to the corneal endothelium and the status

---

Pre-operative assessment

The aims of the hospital pre-operative assessment are to:

- establish the best corrected visual acuity
- confirm the diagnosis of cataract
- exclude coexisting ocular disease
- plan the optical management, in particular biometry
- alert surgeons to potential areas of increased risk
- discuss the procedure with the patient.

of support for the lens. Pre-existing corneal endothelial pathology (e.g. Fuch's dystrophy) or zonular weakness (e.g. pseudoexfoliation) should be highlighted in the referral as both would increase the risk of complications from cataract surgery. Intraocular pressure should be measured prior to pupillary dilatation. During dilated fundus examination one should look out for diabetic retinopathy, ARMD and optic neuropathy, in particular, glaucoma.

Pre-operative medical investigations

Based on the Royal College of Ophthalmologists' *Local Anaesthesia for Intraocular Surgery* guidelines, a patient due to undergo cataract surgery who has no history of significant systemic disease and no abnormal findings on examination at a nurse-led assessment does not require special investigations. Any patient requiring special tests may need a medical opinion.

Key points to consider are:

- **Systemic hypertension** should be controlled well before the patient is scheduled for surgery and not lowered immediately prior to surgery.
- **Angina** should be controlled by a patient's usual angina medication, which should be available in theatre. Every effort should be made to make the experience as stress-free as possible. Generally patients should not have surgery within three months of a myocardial infarct.
- **Diabetic patients** should have their blood sugar controlled. If surgery is planned under local anaesthesia, diabetic patients should have their usual medication and oral intake.
- Patients with **chronic obstructive pulmonary disease** may benefit from an open draping system or high-flow oxygen-enriched air system below the drapes.
- For patients with **valvular heart disease** there is no need for antibiotic prophylaxis for intraocular surgery.
- Patients on **warfarin** should have an international normalized ratio (INR) check (which describes the results of a blood clotting test) prior to surgery (see below).

Medication

Warfarin

The Royal College of Ophthalmologists' guidelines for cataract surgery state that to stop warfarin risks stroke and death; the risk of stroke increases to 1:100. The patient's INR should be checked to ensure that it is within the desired therapeutic range (set by the treating physician), and if needle local anaesthesia is performed the risk of orbital haemorrhage is increased by 0.2–1.0%. Either sub-Tenon's or topical anaesthesia is recommended for these patients.

Aspirin

Aspirin is generally not discontinued prior to cataract surgery.

Flomax

A significant proportion of men aged 60 and older with cataract have benign prostatic hypertrophy (BPH). The BPH drug Flomax (tamsulosin hydrochloride) causes iris complications during phacoemulsification known as intraoperative floppy iris syndrome (IFIS). IFIS describes a floppy iris that billows in response to normal intraocular fluid currents, a strong propensity to iris prolapse and progressive miosis intraoperatively. Complications related to IFIS can be reduced:

- Ask patients before cataract surgery if they are taking Flomax. Discontinuing the drug for two weeks before surgery may lessen the floppiness of the iris, though it will not eliminate it. Any prior history of Flomax use is important because IFIS cases can still occur in those who have discontinued the drug, even one to two years earlier.
- Common techniques such as mechanical pupil stretching or partial thickness sphincterotomies do not appear to work for IFIS.
- Disposable iris retractors (Figure 2.2) or pupil expansion rings are the best way to maintain a larger pupil.

It should be noted that Flomax is prescribed for some women with urinary retention.

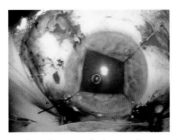

Figure 2.2 Per-operative photograph during phacoemulsification cataract surgery using disposable iris hooks for retraction. Trypan blue (VisionBlue) has been used to stain the anterior capsule to allow capsulorhexis to be easily performed in the absence of a red reflex during surgery.

Pre-operative tests

The tests required prior to cataract surgery are listed in the box below.

Refraction
An accurate pre-operative subjective refraction is vital to ensure that the correct intraocular lens implant is chosen during cataract surgery.

For example, if the patient is highly myopic in both eyes and only has a cataract in one eye, careful discussion with the patient is required in selecting the intraocular lens power for the affected eye. If the operated eye is left emmetropic after surgery (as is normally done in most cases), there is a high risk of post-operative anisometropia. As such, it is usual to aim for

---

Pre-operative tests

- Refraction
- Near and distance visual acuity
- Biometry
- B-scan ultrasonography, if no fundus view obtainable
- Other optional tests—corneal topography, specular microscopy

post-operative low myopia in the operated eye. If the myopic patient has cataract in both eyes, emmetropia is a possible option provided that the second eye is operated on soon after the first. Myopic patients often dislike being left even slightly hypermetropic after cataract surgery. To avoid this it is usual to aim for the patient's postoperative refraction to be slightly myopic.

Near and distance visual acuity

The best corrected visual acuity for near and distance should be obtained. Although Snellen measurements are the most common test for distance acuity, LogMAR visual acuity (Figure 2.3) measurements provide a better and more accurate means of comparing pre- and post-operative visual acuity. It is important to realize that visual acuity measurements are only one test of visual performance. Visual acuity does not always relate to vision in environments with variable lighting conditions, in which glare and pupil constriction may reduce the effective visual acuity.

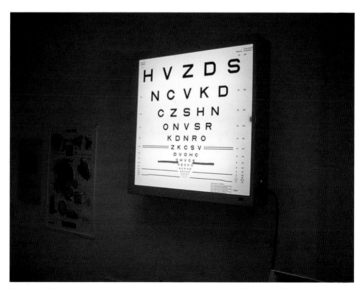

Figure 2.3 Visual acuity chart based on the LogMAR scale

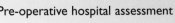
Biometry

Biometry measurements of both eyes are essential prior to cataract surgery. This is normally performed in the hospital by trained nurses, orthoptists or optometrists. Determination of the lens implant power needed to give any desired post-operative refraction requires, at a minimum, measurement of two key variables:

- anterior corneal curvature in two orthogonal meridians, and
- axial length of the eye.

These measurements are then entered into an appropriate formula.

Keratometers measure anterior corneal curvature over a small annular zone (usually between 2 and 4 mm in diameter) and assume this is spherical. Contact lenses should be removed at least 48 hours prior to keratometry because their long-term use can induce a reversible corneal flattening. A variety of manual, automated and hand-held keratometers is available.

The axial length of the eye is measured from the corneal vertex to the fovea and can be measured using either A-mode ultrasound or an optical interferometric technique. The normal axial length of the eye is between 22.0 and 24.5 mm.

The A-mode transducer is commonly 5 mm in diameter and emits short pulses of weakly focused ultrasound at a frequency of 10 MHz. In the intervals between these emissions, echoes are received by the same transducer, which are converted to electric signals and plotted as spikes on a display. The accuracy of measurements obtained by a skilled operator in a regularly shaped eye is generally within 0.1 mm.

An optical interferometer specifically designed for lens implant power calculation is commercially available (IOLMaster; Carl Zeiss) (Figure 2.4). This system is widely used and can measure the axial length, keratometry and anterior chamber depth of the eye. It uses a low coherence Doppler interferometer to measure axial length. In-built formulae allow calculation of lens implant power. Dense cataracts and corneal or vitreous opacities may preclude measurement with this system. The system is a non-contact one and is ideal in terms of patient comfort and compliance. This

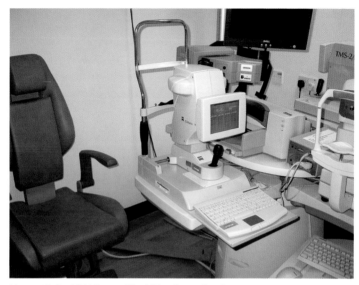

Figure 2.4 IOLMaster (Carl Zeiss), used in biometry measurements prior to cataract surgery

system has proved to be highly accurate and simple to use in a variety of difficult measurement situations.

B-scan ultrasonography
B-scan ultrasonography is useful in eyes with dense cataracts that preclude a visual assessment of the posterior segment. This is to exclude coincidental pathology (e.g. retinal detachment, choroidal tumour) that may be present and which may impact on the post-operative result of cataract surgery.

Other optional tests
Corneal topography can be a useful investigation to show the true shape of the cornea prior to cataract surgery. This can help the surgeon to plan the sites of incisions in cases of high corneal astigmatism, where the surgeon may either operate on the steep corneal meridian or combine the procedure with corneal relaxing

incisions at the site of the steep meridian. This would allow a better post-operative refractive result.

As the corneal endothelium is vulnerable to damage during cataract surgery, it is sometimes useful to document the status of the endothelium with specular microscopy. This assessment has a prognostic value for corneal survival after cataract surgery. In the event that the cornea has a reduced endothelial cell count prior to surgery, the surgeon can counsel the patient appropriately regarding the increased risk of corneal decompensation from cataract surgery.

Presbyopic patients with cataract

With the increasing improvements in cataract surgery techniques and technologies, the demand for a better post-operative result is increasing (e.g. spectacle independence after surgery). As many patients attending for cataract surgery are already in the presbyopic age-group, presbyopic lens exchange, or 'PRELEX', has become a possibility. This allows the patient to be free from the need to use optical correction aids, such as spectacles, for near or distance work after cataract surgery.

PRELEX is now possible due to a combination of factors:

- accurate biometry
- precise and complication-free modern cataract surgery
- reduction of pre-existing astigmatism at the time of cataract surgery
- availability of multifocal and accommodative intraocular lenses.

The ideal patient for PRELEX is a hyperopic presbyope who dislikes wearing glasses and has clinically significant lens changes. The patient must also be able to accept the possible need for glasses in the event of uneventful cataract surgery. The patient must also be aware of the need to adjust to a new visual system and to accept that the ability to have good, unaided near vision may take a period of time to develop. Multifocal and accommodative intraocular lenses are discussed in Chapter 4.

Summary

Cataract is the leading cause of age-related visual loss, and it will only become more common with the increasing life expectancy of our society. Given the magnitude of the associated healthcare burden, an expanded role for the optometrist in patient assessment, preparation and aftercare for cataract surgery is inevitable. As such, it is essential for optometrists to have good knowledge of both the condition and the surgery as integration between ophthalmic healthcare professionals continues.

Further reading

Allan B. (2001). Cataract surgery. Patient preparation and technique. *Optometry Today*, July: 28–33.

Datiles III M.B. and Ansari R.R. (2005). Clinical evaluation of cataracts. In: *Duane's Clinical Ophthalmology*. Ed: Tasman W. and Jaegar E.A. Lippincott, Williams and Wilkins, Chapter 73B.

Howes F (2006). Patient work-up for cataract surgery. In: *Ophthalmology*. Ed: Yanoff M. and Duker J.S. Elsevier, Chapter 43.

The Royal College of Ophthalmologists (2004). *Cataract Surgery Guidelines*. www.rcophth.ac.uk/about/publications.

The Royal College of Anaesthetists and The Royal College of Ophthalmologists. *Local Anaesthesia for Intraocular Surgery (guidelines)*. www.rcophth.ac.uk/about/publications.

Thomson D. (2001). Methods of assessing cataract and the effect of opacities on vision. *Optometry Today*, June: 26–31.

3
Pre-operative biometry and intraocular lens calculation

Sally J Embleton

Introduction

Intraocular lens (IOL) design has evolved in recent years, resulting in more emphasis on the refractive component of cataract surgery. As patients now judge the success of cataract surgery through the post-operative refractive result, it is necessary to minimize post-operative ametropia.

Every aspect of cataract surgery influences the final refractive result, and this chapter will discuss the pre-operative measurements and considerations that play an essential role in optimizing the post-operative refractive outcome. There are, however, a number of surgical factors that will also affect this result. For example, the capsulorhexis should ideally be smaller than the IOL optic, and the viscoelastic should be removed from behind the lens as failure to do this will result in an anterior shift in the IOL position and a post-operative myopic result.

The dioptric power of the IOL implanted is decided upon pre-operatively, and in most cases is chosen so as to leave the patient as near to emmetropia as possible following surgery. The power of the IOL is determined by measuring the power of the cornea and axial length of the eye. The power of the cornea is measured using keratometry or corneal topography and the axial length of the eye is assessed by biometry, of which there are several different methods.

Biometry is not an exact science, being an indirect measure that utilizes either light or sound to calculate the length of the eye. The components of the eye influence the final measurement, and similarly to all physiological variables within the general population these follow a normal distribution. It therefore follows that the post-operative outcome will also tend to follow a similar pattern, albeit with a narrower range of error as techniques improve. It should be noted however that all patients should be counselled prior to surgery and informed of the limitations of this indirect measurement. With all normal distributions there are individuals who lie at the extreme ends and as such will prove more unpredictable in terms of post-operative refractive success.

Refractive error

The refractive error of an eye is determined by four elements:

- The power of the cornea
- The length of the eye
- The anterior chamber depth
- The effective power of the lens (determined by its shape and position in the eye)

These elements can be measured using either keratometry or biometry and can then be applied to a number of different IOL equations. These equations are used to determine the power of the IOL to be implanted (they are discussed in more detail later in this chapter).

Keratometry

Keratometry provides a measurement of the anterior curvature of the central 3 mm corneal diameter, although this area does vary between instruments. The measure of curvature is used to determine the power of the cornea, and in order to calculate this the refractive index of the cornea is required. This is assumed by the machine and can differ between instruments, with the range used being between 1.3315 and 1.3380. This variation may appear to be a potential problem when conducting biometry. However, it is not the values used that are important but that consistency is maintained in the machines being used and their values within a department.

Keratometry values can be depicted in either dioptric form or in terms of radius of curvature, measured in millimetres. When conducting keratometry to calculate IOL power, corneal curvature is usually expressed in terms of dioptric power. Two values are obtained from keratometry, and these values are typically 90 degrees from one another. Most individuals have a degree of corneal astigmatism, very few have truly spherical corneas. If there is no difference in these numbers the individual has no corneal astigmatism. If a discrepancy exists between these numbers, with the larger of the two being at the vertical orientation, the patient is said to have with-the-rule astigmatism and if the horizontal meridian has the higher power then they have against-the-rule astigmatism. If the axis lies between 30 and 60 and 120 and 150 degrees then they have oblique astigmatism. In the vast majority of individuals the meridians are found to lie 90 degrees apart, and in these instances regular astigmatism exists. Patients with corneal disorders such as keratoconus are often said to have irregular astigmatism and in such cases the principal meridians lie less than 90 degrees from one another.

Errors in keratometry

The cornea is the most powerful focusing part of the eye, accounting for two-thirds of the refractive power, with 98% of the population having a corneal power between 40 and 48 D. Of these, 68% have a power between 42 and 45 D. Accurate keratometry is essential when determining the correct power of an IOL, but there are a number of factors that can lead to inaccuracies in measurement, as follows.

Diurnal variations in corneal physiology
The refractive index of the cornea has been shown to exhibit diurnal fluctuations, and it has been found that these variations in density are related to corneal hydration. It is not feasible to measure the refractive index of every individual cornea and as a result an average value is assumed, as detailed above. The majority of individuals will have a corneal refractive index near to this value, but significant deviations from this may result in post-operative refractive surprises that can not be predicted nor controlled for.

Contact lens wearers
A contact lens can result in alterations in the curvature of a patient's cornea. Patients should be instructed to cease wearing contact lenses prior to their pre-operative appointment in order

to ensure stability of corneal parameters. A period of two weeks for soft contact lenses and four weeks for rigid contact lenses should suffice but stability of corneal curvature measurements between visits is strongly recommended to confirm this as this can vary between individuals.

Non-sphericity of the cornea

A keratometer makes a number of assumptions when obtaining measures of corneal curvature. One assumption is that the cornea is spherical in nature, which we know not to be the case. The cornea flattens towards its periphery, and the rate in which it flattens differs between individuals. A keratometer provides a measure of corneal curvature from the central 3 mm; therefore the likelihood for error is greater for a person in whom the rate of flattening is relatively high. It is also important that the patient is viewing the target to assume measurement of the cornea along the visual axis (slightly nasal and inferior to the geometric centre of the eye). Incorrect positioning of the mires can result in measurement of the cornea in the wrong area, with subsequent errors in IOL calculation.

Improper calibration

Steel balls of known curvature are used to calibrate manual keratometers. These should be used routinely to ensure accurate measurement of curvature, and hence power.

Failure to focus eyepieces

It is important that in manual keratometry the eyepieces are focused correctly, in accordance with the observer's refractive error. This ensures accommodation is not stimulated, which can result in erroneous measurements. The eyepieces are focused by turning them anticlockwise and then slowly turning them clockwise until the mires are in sharp focus.

Inadequate tear film

In some instances it is not possible to acquire a good image of the mires due to disruptions of the corneal surface, either due to corneal scarring or to insufficiencies in the tear film. In such cases artificial tears of low viscosity (so as not to significantly affect readings) can be used, and in the majority of cases this provides a stable surface for the subsequent measurement of corneal curvature.

Previous refractive surgery

Refractive corneal laser surgery results in changes in the relationship between the curvature of the anterior and posterior surfaces of the cornea. Keratometry measurements on patients who have had previous corneal refractive surgery (e.g. LASIK) will be higher than the true value of the corneal power. If this value is then used to calculate the IOL power, the patient will end up hypermetropic post-operatively.

Although there are many methods to determine the corneal power following refractive surgery, one way in which a reasonably accurate measurement of corneal power can be extrapolated is by using the clinical history method. It is necessary to have details of the patient's keratometry measurements and their spectacle prescription prior to the refractive procedure, and their post-operative manifest refraction prior to the development of any lenticular opacity. In this method the difference between the spherical equivalent of the patient's refraction pre and post refractive surgery is derived. This difference is then deducted from the patient's pre-operative mean keratometric value to provide a new corneal power that can be used to determine the power of the IOL. For example:

Pre refractive surgery refraction	−3.00 DS
Pre refractive surgery keratometry	average 43 D
Post refractive surgery refraction	−0.50 DS
Change in refraction	−2.50 DS
New keratometry reading	40.5 D

A comprehensive summary of techniques for determining the corneal power following myopic LASIK is provided at *www.doctor-hill.com/iol-main/lasik.htm*.

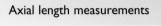

Axial length measurements

Most eyes (approximately 96%) have an axial length between 21 and 25.5 mm, and the majority of these (60%) lie within 22.5 and 24.5 mm. Provided there is no significant difference in refractive errors between eyes it is very unlikely for a patient to have an inter-eye axial length difference of 0.3 mm or more. Measurements that fall outside these parameters should be viewed with caution and evidence for their anomaly sought.

The length of the eye can be assessed using either light (partial coherence interferometry—PCI) or sound (A-scan ultrasonography). In addition, A-scan ultrasonography can be further divided into contact and immersion biometry (with the use of a Prager shell, as outlined below). The various ways in which axial length can be measured is discussed in full below.

Partial coherence interferometry

Optical biometry benefits from being quick, non-invasive, requiring no uncomfortable topical anaesthesia, and having excellent repeatability between different users. Its one disadvantage is that measurements are difficult, or impossible, to obtain on patients with very dense cataracts or significant corneal scarring. In such cases it is necessary to resort to using A-scan ultrasound biometry.

PCI is conducted using the Zeiss IOLMaster (*see* Figure 2.4), which was introduced in Europe in 1999.

The IOLMaster is a non-contact biometer that provides consistent measurements, within ±0.02 mm. This is approximately a fivefold increase in the accuracy of axial length measurements when compared with ultrasound biometry. The advent of the IOLMaster thus enabled a significant improvement to the pre-operative assessment of patients undergoing cataract surgery. In addition to axial length, the machine can be used to provide measurements of corneal curvature, anterior chamber depth and 'white-to-white' (the corneal diameter).

Interferometry works on the principle of constructive and destructive interference. Two waves that coincide in phase are additive (constructive) while two waves out of phase cancel one another out (destructive). The IOLMaster utilizes a modified Michelson interferometer to obtain measurements of the distance travelled, or length. This comprises two infrared light beams with a wavelength of 780 nm, a detector, two mirrors and a semitransparent mirror or beam splitter (Figure 3.1).

The IOLMaster provides a measurement from the corneal vertex to the retinal pigment epithelium, unlike the A-scan ultrasound biometer, which measures from the corneal vertex to the internal limiting membrane (between the vitreous and retina). This represents a 0.2 to 0.3 mm difference between the two techniques, which is equivalent to the thickness of the retina at the macula. During its calibration process the measurements acquired with the IOLMaster were compared with those made using high-resolution immersion biometry (Grieshaber Biometric System), which is able to measure with an accuracy of ±20 μm. Based on this comparison an internal algorithm was incorporated

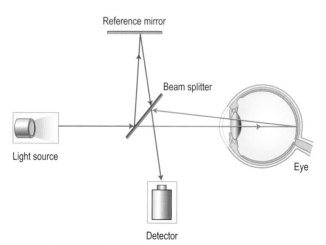

Figure 3.1 Schematic of the IOLMaster interferometer

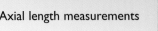

into the IOLMaster so that its axial length measurement is identical to that of the high-resolution Grieshaber Biometric System.

Useful principles for axial length acquisition

As already detailed, the IOLMaster is a non-contact procedure and thus no corneal anaesthesia is required when acquiring measurements. The patient is seated at the machine with their chin on the chin-rest and forehead against the upper bar (comparable to a slit lamp) and is instructed to look at the red fixation light to ensure measurement along the visual axis. The reflection of the fixation light needs to be correctly centred within the circle, although sharp focusing of the light is not necessary.

A precautionary safety mechanism is incorporated into the machine so that the number of axial length measures taken in any one session is limited to 20 per eye. This limits the amount of laser light a patient is exposed to and ensures that the exposure does not exceed recommended levels.

A number of scans should be acquired by the operator, and should any one of these differ by more than 0.2 mm the machine will not calculate the mean value and an 'evaluation' error message will be displayed. In such a scenario the scans should be examined and edited, and if necessary, additional measurements taken so that the standard deviation is kept to a minimum. It is good practice to ensure you have five consistent measurements prior to calculating the IOL implant power.

In every scan acquired the signal-to-noise ratio (SNR) is given, which provides an indication of the quality of the resultant scan. On the printout, the scan with the highest SNR is arrowed. An ideal scan will have an SNR above 5.0 (Figure 3.2) and a good scan will have an SNR greater than 2.0 (Figure 3.3). Scans with an SNR between 1.6 and 2.0 (Figure 3.4) will be marked with an exclamation mark and an evaluation of the scan is recommended. These may well be valid and usable scans, however, and should not necessarily be discarded.

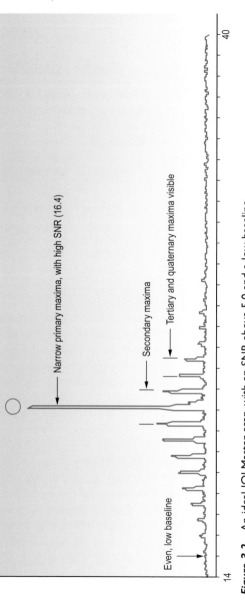

Figure 3.2 An ideal IOLMaster scan, with an SNR above 5.0 and a low baseline

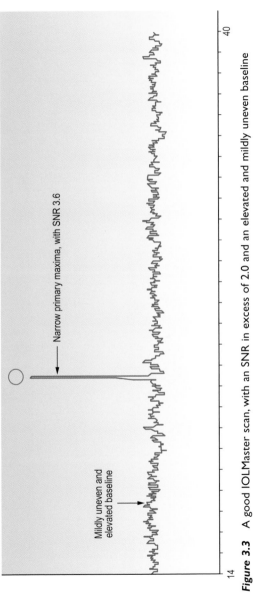

Narrow primary maxima, with SNR 3.6

Mildly uneven and
elevated baseline

Figure 3.3 A good IOLMaster scan, with an SNR in excess of 2.0 and an elevated and mildly uneven baseline

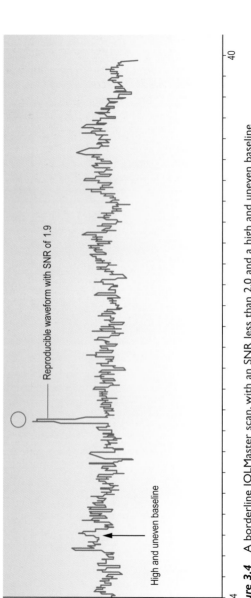

Reproducible waveform with SNR of 1.9

High and uneven baseline

Figure 3.4 A borderline IOLMaster scan, with an SNR less than 2.0 and a high and uneven baseline

The SNR is determined by the amount of light received by the detector and hence the density of the lenticular opacity. The higher the SNR the better the quality of the received signal; this can be seen visually on the resultant scan, with the baseline being low and even (Figure 3.2). As the SNR decreases, the baseline elevates and becomes increasingly more uneven (Figures 3.3 and 3.4).

For a measurement of axial length from the IOLMaster to be deemed acceptable it is necessary that the main peak is clearly distinguishable from the baseline, and at least four repeatable scans are acquired. In scans where the SNR is less than 1.6 it is difficult to distinguish the primary maxima and an error message will be depicted by the machine. In such cases it may be necessary to resort to A-scan ultrasonography.

It is worth noting that close inspection of scans that deviate from the average value is advisable. This can be done by taking the mouse cursor to the baseline beneath the white spot and clicking the left mouse button. This will confirm that the primary maxima has a sharp central point rather than being double-spiked in nature (Figure 3.5). A double-spiked peak occurs when light is reflected back at both the internal limiting membrane (left-hand spike) and retinal pigment epithelium (right-hand spike) layers of the retina. If the marker is placed at the retinal pigment epithelium layer spike the scan is acceptable, but where the marker lies at the site of the internal limiting layer it is advisable to repeat the scan rather than to realign the marker manually. In addition a double spike can also occur when reflection of the light occurs at both the retinal pigment epithelium and choroidal layers. In such cases the choroidal peak will be positioned on the right-hand side and the resultant axial length will be significantly longer than the others obtained. Movement of the gate to the retinal epithelium layer peak will result in adjustment of the axial length measure, which should then be comparable with the others taken.

Practical advice for the IOL Master

In cases where there is difficulty in obtaining scans with an acceptable SNR the operator can consider changing the position

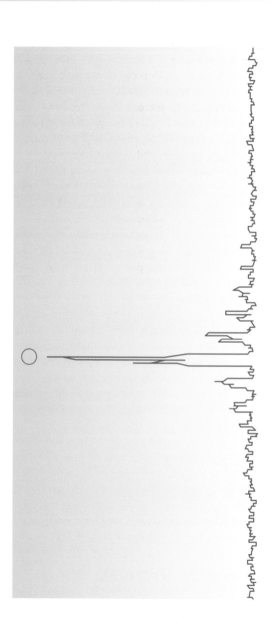

Figure 3.5 An IOLMaster scan with the primary maxima having a double-spike peak

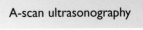

that the scans are being taken from. The patient will initially be seated correctly and the fixation light positioned centrally. This can be altered so that the light is placed at any position within the 12, 3, 6 and 9 o'clock areas, with the reflection placed at the inner edge of the circle. In addition, the distance between the patient and the machine can be increased by pulling the joystick back. This will result in the light reflection becoming defocused, with it filling the entire circle. Provided the SNRs are acceptable and the scans are repeatable and within the accepted deviation, these axial length readings can be used to determine the power of the IOL to be implanted.

In patients with dry eyes it may be necessary to instil artificial tears prior to acquisition (tear substitutes of low viscosity are advisable), and in these patients it is common that the resultant scans have poor SNRs. In most instances dry eye patients will only prove problematic when attempting to acquire consistent keratometry measures with the IOLMaster.

Patients who have problems with fixation can wear their spectacles, and in cases of high ametropia this is advisable, provided the lens material is not tinted. However, wearing contact lenses will result in a reduction in the SNR during axial length measurement and erroneous keratometry values, and therefore should be removed prior to the pre-operative biometry appointment.

A-scan ultrasonography

Ultrasound is defined as being sound with a frequency more than 20 kHz. In A-scan ultrasound biometry a frequency of 10 MHz is used, which enables restricted penetration of the sound beam with adequate resolution of the internal structures. Lower frequencies result in greater penetration of tissue, and higher frequencies result in better resolution but less penetration.

A beam of sound is directed through the eye, and reflections of the sound waves travel back towards the probe at every interface, where they are recorded. The sound beam is generated by piezoelectric crystals within the ultrasound probe or transducer. A piezoelectric material has the ability to generate a voltage in response to applied mechanical stress. These crystals are placed within the transducer of an ultrasound machine, where they act as both sensors and actuators. An electric current is applied to the piezoelectric crystal, causing it to flex and to produce a sound wave that is directed through the eye. A proportion of the sound wave is reflected back to the transducer at every interface between materials of differing density, with the remainder being transmitted through the remaining structures. In the case of the eye, the main reflections occur at the waterbath–anterior corneal interface (in the case of immersion ultrasound only), the posterior corneal–aqueous humor interface, the aqueous humor–anterior crystalline lens interface, the posterior crystalline lens–vitreous interface and the vitreous–retinal interface. At each of these points the sound reflected back to the transducer causes the piezoelectric crystals to flex, producing an electrical signal. These signals, known as 'echoes', are sent to an oscilloscope, where they can be visualized; this visual representation is called an echogram.

The amplitude of an echo is determined by the tissue types of the structures and the angle at which the sound beam hits them. Maximum amplitude will be seen where the difference in density between the two interfaces is at a maximum and when the beam reaches these structures at right angles. This is how this type of biometry gets its name: the 'A' in A-scan refers to 'amplitude' as the resultant scans are two-dimensional in nature and it is the distances between the major spikes at each of the interfaces that are used to obtain a measurement of axial length.

In A-scan ultrasound the resultant axial length obtained is not a direct measurement. The machine measures the time it takes for the sound beam to travel from one interface to the next. The distance is determined by multiplying this value with constant values for the speed of sound in varying media of differing densities.

Sound travels faster through solids than liquids, and faster through liquids than air. In most modern A-scan biometers constant values are used for the speed of sound through the cornea and lens (1641 m/s) and aqueous and vitreous (1532 m/s). These values are only averages, however, and the actual values will vary between subjects, thus highlighting a limitation of this technique in acquiring measurements of axial length. For instance, the density of the crystalline lens does not remain static throughout life but increases with age. This means that the speed at which sound travels through this structure will also increase over time, and unless compensated for by the A-scan biometer it will result in small inaccuracies. Modern machines (Ocuscan RxP; Alcon Laboratories) incorporate age-compensation software, which changes the speed of sound through the crystalline lens according to the patient's age, thus improving reliability.

Sources of error using A-scan ultrasonography

A biometric error of as little as 1 mm will result in a post-operative refractive error of up to 3 D. In its biometry guidelines in 2001, the Royal College of Ophthalmologists suggested that 50% of patients should have a post-operative outcome within 0.5 D of the target refraction, 90% within 1 D and 99% within 2 D.

Corneal compression
There are two methods of conducting A-scan ultrasonography: contact and immersion. With contact ultrasonography the probe is in direct contact with the eye, as shown in Figure 3.6.

In immersion ultrasonography (Figure 3.7) the transducer probe is held in a plastic shell known as a Prager shell. This shell has a diameter greater than that of the cornea and as such sits on the rigid sclera. Once the shell is in place on the eye saline can be injected through the disposable tubing so that the transducer is immersed in a water bath. This means that there is no contact between the eye and the probe. However, similarly to contact ultrasonography, corneal anaesthesia is required to ensure patient comfort.

Immersion ultrasonography is technically more difficult to conduct than the contact technique. Previously it was necessary

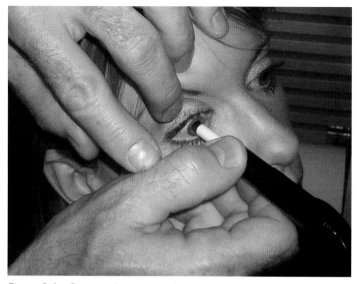

Figure 3.6 Contact ultrasonography

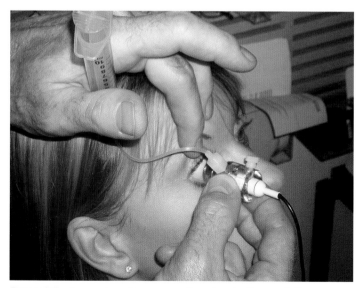

Figure 3.7 Immersion ultrasonography using the Prager shell

for patients to adopt a horizontal position during immersion ultrasound, thus restricting its use in ophthalmology outpatient clinics. More recently, developments in the Prager shell design have meant that immersion ultrasonography can now be conducted with patients in the upright position. However, it can still be a messy procedure, and patients should be warned in advance that water is involved and they may get a little wet.

The major advantage of immersion biometry is that it eliminates errors caused by corneal compression. The cornea is a deformable structure, and when exposed to any degree of pressure it will depress, shortening the anterior chamber. Even for the most experienced of users contact ultrasonography will result in a reduction in axial length of 0.1 to 0.3 mm. Improvements in design, such as spring loaded probes, have been introduced in an attempt to address this potential source of error, but they do not eliminate the problem entirely and should therefore be used with caution. The average anterior chamber depth is 3.24 mm, and this is known to reduce with advancing age as the crystalline lens increases in size. When the anterior chamber depth is measured as being significantly less than the average (even if the echogram looks adequate) the scan should be viewed with caution and measurements repeated. Another check that can be used is to compare the measurements from both eyes. In the absence of anisometropia it is unusual for there to be an axial length difference of more than 0.3 mm between the two eyes and the anterior depth of both eyes should be similar. An axial length measurement that is falsely short will result in the indicated IOL power being higher than necessary and the patient will have a post-operative myopic result.

Interpretation of the echogram

Figure 3.8 shows an ideal scan for immersion ultrasonography. The resultant echogram comprises five spikes: anterior cornea (C1), posterior cornea (C2), anterior lens (L1), posterior lens (L2) and retina (R). This is different to a contact ultrasound echogram, where only four spikes result (C, L1, L2, and R) due to the corneal contact with the probe. In immersion ultrasonography the probe sits away from the cornea and is

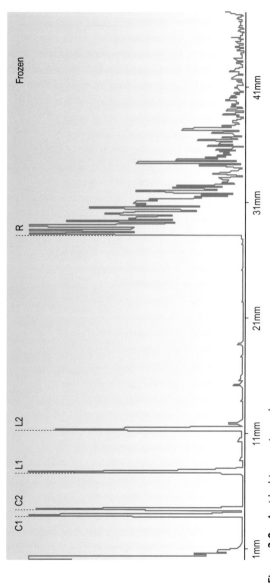

Figure 3.8 An ideal immersion echogram

separated from it by fluid; the extra spike seen in an immersion echogram results from the water bath–anterior corneal interface. The remaining four spikes refer to the posterior corneal surface, the anterior and posterior crystalline lens and the retina. At each of these spikes the A-scan ultrasound machine places a gate (in this case a dotted line), which indicates where the machine is taking the measurements to and hence what velocities it is using for the calculation of each section of the eye. The echoes visualized posterior to the scleral spike are due to reflection of the sound beam from the orbital fat layers.

Correct interpretation of the echogram is essential in ensuring correct alignment of the probe and correct measurement of the length of the eye from the corneal apex to the macula, i.e. along the visual axis.

Visual axis alignment

If the sound beam does not travel along the visual axis the resultant axial length reading will be falsely short and the IOL power calculated will be higher than is required, resulting in a myopic post-operative refractive error. In order to determine whether the sound beam has travelled along the correct axis it is necessary to examine the crystalline lens spikes. If the alignment is incorrect the posterior lens spike will be significantly longer or shorter than the anterior lens spike. This occurs because the sound beam does not reach the anterior lens surface perpendicularly and therefore much of the reflected sound from this surface does not travel back to the probe, resulting in a reduced amplitude signal and hence a reduced spike. In ideal alignment of the probe the posterior spike will be slightly shorter than the anterior lens spike (Figure 3.9). If, however, the posterior spike is significantly shorter (Figure 3.10) or significantly longer (Figure 3.11) than the anterior spike, the sound beam is misaligned and the echogram should be discarded.

Probe perpendicularity

It is important that the probe sits on the cornea perpendicularly to ensure the sound beam is directed along the eye at right

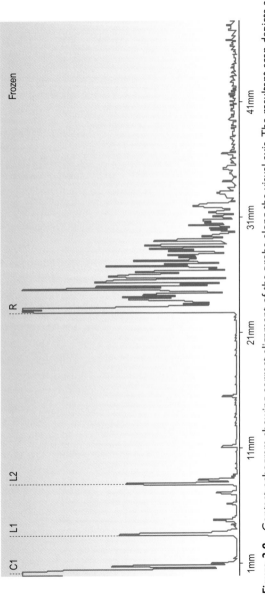

Figure 3.9 Contact echogram showing correct alignment of the probe along the visual axis. The resultant scan depicts a posterior lens spike that is slightly shorter than the anterior lens spike

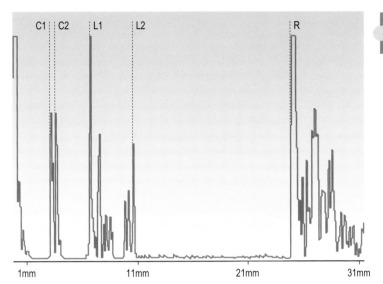

Figure 3.10 Immersion echogram showing improper alignment of the probe, with it failing to align along the visual axis. The resultant scan has a posterior lens spike significantly shorter than the anterior spike

angles to the retina. Poor alignment will result in an echogram that has a sloping retinal spike, and incorrect positioning of the retinal gate will ensue (Figure 3.12). This will result in a measurement that is artificially long, with the IOL power calculated being weaker than is required. The patient will end up post-operatively in the worst-case scenario, being hypermetropic, and not only having reduced distance vision but also being unable to read without spectacles. Perpendicularity can be confirmed when both the retinal and scleral spikes are of high amplitude and the retinal spike rises steeply from baseline with no sloping or jagged steps on the ascending portion (Figure 3.13).

Optic nerve misalignment
As already indicated, it is important that the sound beam travels along the visual axis to the macula. If the sound beam travels

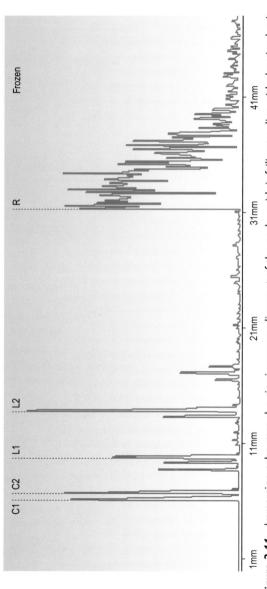

Figure 3.11 Immersion echogram showing improper alignment of the probe, with it failing to align with the visual axis. The resultant scan has a posterior lens spike significantly longer than the anterior spike

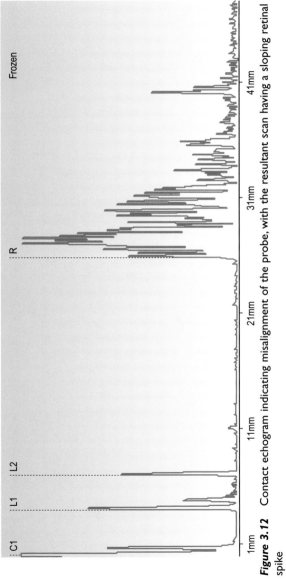

Figure 3.12 Contact echogram indicating misalignment of the probe, with the resultant scan having a sloping retinal spike

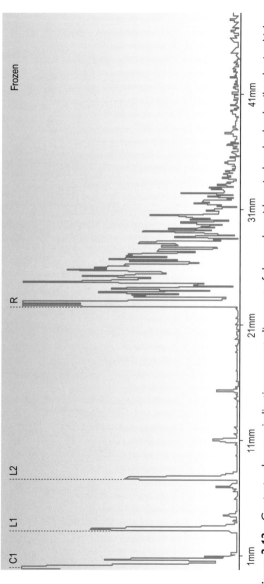

Figure 3.13 Contact echogram indicating correct alignment of the probe with retinal and scleral spikes having high amplitude and the retinal spike rising steeply

along the optic nerve head the resultant scan will be erroneously short, and the patient will have a post-operative myopic result. Misalignment of the probe along the optic nerve is easily recognized; the resultant scan will be devoid of any reflections from the orbital fat (Figure 3.14). In such cases the scan must be repeated.

Dense lenticular opacities

Patients with particularly dense lenticular opacities are not only problematic to the IOLMaster, but also require closer attention by the biometrist using A-scan ultrasonography, in terms of gain and correct placement of gates.

The gain of an ultrasound machine can be compared to the volume of a stereo. Increasing it will result in better penetration of the sound beam through the dense opacity (compare to listening to a stereo from a different room) but poorer resolution (compare to reductions in the clarity of the bass). If the gain is set too high the resultant peaks on the echogram will have flat tops and resolution of the interfaces that lie close to one another (for instance the retina and sclera) will be less clearly defined. In such instances it will be more difficult to interpret whether the sound beam travelled along the visual axis because the heights of the lens spikes at every interface are at a maximum (Figure 3.15). Conversely, if the gain is set too low the retinal spike will be of reduced amplitude, or in some instances almost absent (Figure 3.16). Setting the gain too low for adequate visualization of the retinal spike can result in incorrect placement of the retinal gate at the scleral interface, which will result in an error of up to 1 mm. In such cases the eye will be measured as being artificially long, with an IOL of insufficient power being implanted. The result is a post-operative hypermetropic refraction, with the patient having neither functional distance nor near vision without correction. Care should be employed so that the gain is set to allow adequate penetration with greatest resolution, thus ensuring the resultant scans are of the optimum quality.

Every A-scan biometer uses internal algorithms. Each scan has its initial spike at the anterior or posterior corneal surface (depending upon whether the operator is using the contact or

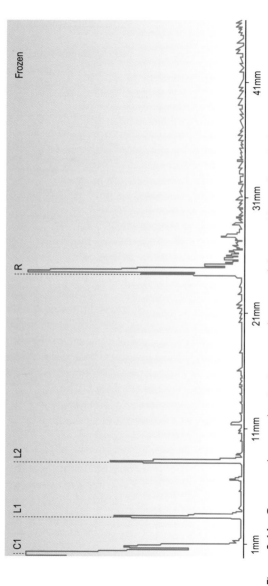

Figure 3.14 Contact echogram showing incorrect alignment of the sound beam through the optic nerve. Reflections from the orbital fat are absent

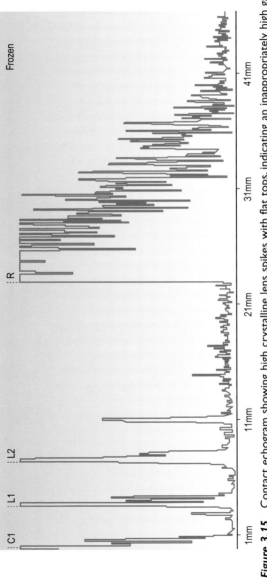

Figure 3.15 Contact echogram showing high crystalline lens spikes with flat tops, indicating an inappropriately high gain

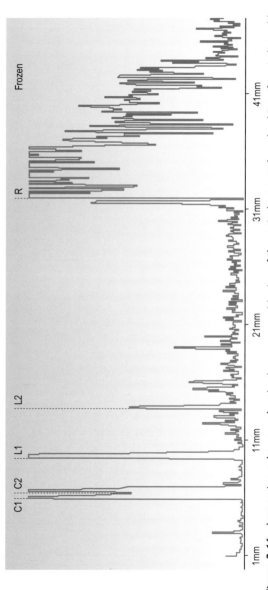

Figure 3.16 Immersion echogram showing improper positioning of the retinal gate at the scleral interface, indicated by the very small retinal spike

immersion technique) and the biometer will look for the second sound reflection or echo at a predetermined distance from the first. It is therefore essential that the biometrist ensures the gates have been assigned correctly on the resultant scan as different velocities are used to calculate the lengths for different sections of the eye. The velocity through the anterior chamber (distance between posterior corneal spike and anterior lens spike) is usually taken as being 1532 m/s, the velocity through the lens (distance between anterior lens spike and posterior lens spike) as being 1641 m/s, and the velocity through the posterior chamber (distance between posterior lens spike and retinal lens spike) as being 1532 m/s, similarly to the anterior chamber. The calculated lengths of each of these sections are then added together to provide an axial length measure.

Incorrect placement of the gates can occur when a patient presents with an extremely dense cataract. A dense lenticular opacity can result in multiple echoes within the crystalline lens matrix due to changes in the density of the lens matter, and in some cases the posterior lens gate may be incorrectly aligned along one of the spikes within the lens nucleus (Figure 3.17). This is less likely to occur with modern A-scan biometers due to improvements in echogram algorithms, but in cases where this error occurs it is necessary for the biometrist to realign the gates correctly. Failure to do this will result in an erroneously thin lens thickness and a falsely long axial length.

A minimum of three good-quality scans should be acquired, and the standard deviation between these scans should be no more than 0.15 mm and ideally less than 0.1 mm. When assessing scans for their quality, look for the following characteristics:

- four or five (depending upon the technique being used) clearly identifiable spikes
- crystalline spikes, with the posterior lens spike being of similar height or slightly shorter than the anterior lens spike
- retinal spike that has a steeply rising configuration
- detectable scleral spike
- correctly positioned gates.

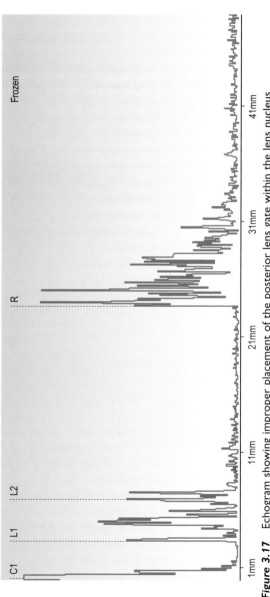

Figure 3.17 Echogram showing improper placement of the posterior lens gate within the lens nucleus

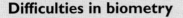

Difficulties in biometry

Posterior staphyloma

Posterior staphyloma is a condition that can be present in highly myopic individuals with long axial lengths. It is caused by elongation of the globe due to thinning and bulging of the sclera and results in an irregular configuration of the retina at the posterior pole.

Posterior staphyloma should be considered in patients with long axial lengths and inconsistencies in axial length measures within and between eyes. Most staphyloma lie in the peripapillary region next to the macula. In cases where the fovea lies on the sloping wall of the staphyloma a small change in direction of the sound beam will result in a large difference in axial length measure. B-scans can be used to diagnose the condition, but difficulties lie in identifying the exact positioning of the fovea and hence the axial length measure that should be used to calculate the power of the IOL. Wherever possible the IOLMaster should be used because accurate measurements of axial length can be acquired using this technique, as long as the patient has adequate fixation.

Silicone oil

Patients who have had a retinal detachment may have undergone a vitrectomy and had silicone oil implanted in the posterior chamber to prevent further detachment. It is common for these patients to develop secondary cataract as a direct result of the retinal detachment surgery. Silicone oil is significantly less dense than the original vitreous gel and therefore sound travels through it much more slowly. Using the standard settings on an ultrasound machine will result in gross overestimation of the patient's eyes length, and if used will render the patient hypermetropic post-operatively. Similarly to patients with posterior staphyloma, patients with silicone oil should whenever possible have measures of axial length conducted using the IOLMaster as this has a setting for silicone oil. In instances where this is not possible it is necessary to correct the IOL power calculated accordingly, or to wait until the silicone oil is removed. It is now common practice to carry out biometry before injection of silicone oil in order to avoid subsequent errors in biometry.

Choosing the appropriate target refraction

In most instances the IOL of choice will either render the patient emmetropic, enabling clear distance vision but necessitating near vision correction for reading, or myopic, for patients who would prefer to be without spectacles when conducting near vision tasks (in the case of monofocal IOLs).

There are a number of factors that must be taken into account when determining the strength of the IOL to be implanted. If cataract surgery is only planned for one eye, it is important not to leave the patient with an intolerable degree of anisometropia. In such cases correction through spectacle wear may be intolerable, either due to aniseikonia (differences in image size) or differential prismatic effects.

Convex lenses result in image magnification while concave lenses cause image minification. Small differences in image size between the two eyes are easily overcome by patients, but when the difference in refraction exceeds 3 or 4 D, binocular fusion is disrupted and wearing the full correction is intolerable.

The tolerance to differential prism is significantly lower, and this must be considered in patients who wear either bifocal or varifocal lenses. Prentice's rule states that the prismatic effect is equal to the power of the lens multiplied by the distance from the optical centre in centimetres. During near vision tasks a bifocal wearer adopts a position in which their line of sight travels through the lens approximately 1 cm below the optical centre. Each dioptre of vertical power difference results in a prismatic effect of 1 Δ. A differential vertical prism of around 1.5 Δ can be tolerated by most individuals, with increases in this resulting in vertical diplopia and spectacle intolerance. In such cases it is necessary for patients to have separate spectacles for distance and for reading. Alternatively they can have a custom-made bifocal known as a 'slab-off', which balances out the differential prism between the two eyes.

Consider the following example, where right cataract surgery is planned:

Right eye: +6.00
Mean sphere: +6.00
Power vertically (1 cm below OC):
   6 Δ Base up

Left eye: +6.00/−2.00 × 180
Mean sphere: +5.00
4 Δ Base up

Note

Both the spherical and cylindrical components of the patient's prescription must be considered. Remember that the maximum vertical effect of a cylinder occurs when its axis is at 180 degrees (with no effect at 90 degrees), thus it follows that the vertical prismatic power of the following prescriptions are:

a. +6.00/−2.00 × 180   = 4 Δ i.e. subtract all of cylinder from sphere

b. +6.00/−2.00 × 45 or 135 = 5 Δ i.e. subtract half of cylinder from sphere

c. +6.00/−2.00 × 90   = 6 Δ i.e. subtract no cylinder from sphere

---

If it is planned to leave the patient emmetropic, the patient would be left with a differential prismatic effect of 4 Δ Base Up—an intolerable amount. If, however, it was planned to leave the patient with 2.5 D of hypermetropia in the right eye, the patient would have 1.5 Δ differential vertical prism, which is likely to be tolerated by the patient.

The target refraction given on the biometry printout refers to the mean sphere and takes no account of the cylindrical element of the cornea. Placing the surgical incision along the steepest meridian of the cornea results in flattening of this profile and a reduction in the degree of corneal astigmatism. The astigmatism present in a patient's pre-operative pair of spectacles is often different to the corneal astigmatism measured using keratometry; this is due to the role the lenticular profile (lenticular astigmatism) plays. Once the crystalline lens is removed, however, it is the corneal astigmatism that influences the amount of cylindrical power required to optimize vision. If the amount of cylindrical power in a patient's spectacles changes significantly with surgery, or is at a different orientation, it can result in difficulties in adaptation and therefore patient dissatisfaction with the procedure. It is therefore important to consider the regularity of the corneal profile prior to surgery, and to work to minimize or prevent further changes in the astigmatism present.

IOL power equations

There are two different types of IOL calculations: regression and theoretical. Regression formulae are based on retrospective analysis of actual post-operative refractive data, and most of these are now obsolete (SRK I and SRK II). Theoretical equations are based on geometric optics as applied to schematic eye models, and these equations attempt to estimate where the effective lens position lies, for greater accuracy in determining the IOL power.

Whatever IOL equation is chosen, a number of variables are required in order to calculate the power of the IOL. These include measures of corneal power (keratometry) and axial length. In addition to this, an IOL equation constant is required. The names given to IOL constants differ for different equations (Table 3.1), and their values are dependent upon the IOL type. Factors such as optic design, haptic angulation and IOL material all play a part in determining this value.

Table 3.1 **IOL constants utilized by various IOL equations**

IOL equation	IOL constant
SRK-T	A constant
Hoffer Q	ACD factor
Holladay 1	Surgeon factor
Holladay 2	ACD factor
Haigis	a0, a1 and a2

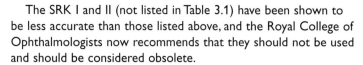

The SRK I and II (not listed in Table 3.1) have been shown to be less accurate than those listed above, and the Royal College of Ophthalmologists now recommends that they should not be used and should be considered obsolete.

The values of the IOL constants are provided by lens manufacturers, having been determined in a laboratory setting. They should be considered as a starting point, with the recommendation being that they are customized or personalized using post-operative refractive data in order to improve surgical outcomes. The constant provided is only valid for contact ultrasonography. For immersion biometry and partial coherence interferometry the value must be increased. Constants for immersion biometry will be higher due to the absence of corneal compression, and in the case of the 'A constant' will be approximately 0.3 units higher. For partial coherence interferometry using the IOLMaster the constants will, once again, be higher. In the case of the A constant the value is typically 0.4 units higher for the IOLMaster. IOLMaster constants for all the IOL equations for most currently available IOLs can be found on the ULIB's (User Group for Laser Interference Biometry) website (www.augenklinik.uni-wuerzburg.de/eulib/const.htm), which can also be accessed through a very useful website devised by Dr Warren Hill (www.doctor-hill.com/physicians/physician_main.htm).

The choice of IOL equation for calculation of the implant power should be chosen by the surgeon, and guidelines for when the various equations should be used are provided by the governing bodies. The Royal College of Ophthalmologists recommends the use of third-generation formulae, with the length of the patient's eye determining what equation should be used (Table 3.2).

IOL equation constants can be customized or personalized by an individual surgeon to optimize post-operative refractive outcomes. Programs for refining these constants can be found on the IOLMaster and on many of the modern A-scan biometers, such as the Ocuscan RxP (Alcon Laboratories). These programs require post-operative refractive data from at least 20 subjects in addition to the IOL type and target refraction. Personalization

Table 3.2 **Recommendations from the Royal College of Ophthalmologists' 2004** *Cataract Surgery Guidelines* **for the choice of IOL equation from axial length**

Axial length (mm)	Recommended IOL equation
<22.0	Hoffer Q/SRK-T
22.0–24.5	SRK-T/Holladay, Haigis
>24.6	SRK-T

should ideally be carried out for each individual surgeon, provided all the pre-operative variables remain unchanged (changes in the type of biometer or keratometer used or a new operative warrant new personalization). It should be noted, however, that although this process will prove effective in the majority of cases it does not eliminate the inherent limits of the IOL equations themselves. The IOL equations outlined so far assume the effective lens position (distance between cornea and lens) according to the patient's axial length. The SRK-T, Holladay 1 and Hoffer Q all assume that short eyes have more shallow anterior chambers and long eyes have deeper anterior chambers. This has been proved to be incorrect, with the majority of eyes having normal anterior chamber depth independent of their length. It therefore follows that using these formulae for patients with particularly long or short axial lengths but normal anterior chamber depths will result in an incorrectly powered IOL being implanted and a post-operative refractive error for the patient.

New IOL equations have been developed more recently. These include the Haigis and Holladay 2 formulae. These equations provide more accurate results in eyes that are of shorter or longer length than average. The Holladay 2 formula works by improving the prediction of the effective lens position, and requires the additional input of anterior chamber depth, corneal diameter (white-to-white), lens thickness, spectacle prescription and patient age. The Haigis formula similarly aims to improve the predicted effective lens position, but in addition it considers the individual geometry of the IOL selection. This equation uses three constants, a0, a1 and a2: a0 works similarly to constants for other IOL equations by moving the prediction curve up or down, a1 is related to the anterior chamber depth and a2 to the axial length.

Summary

As surgical procedures improve, post-operative risks decrease and IOL designs develop, patient expectations increase. Patient satisfaction is largely determined by the post-operative refractive result, and in the majority of cases post-operative emmetropia is desired. This outcome is more attainable if accurate biometry is undertaken, since small errors in axial length measures will result in significant post-operative refractive errors. Advances in the accuracy of axial length measurements have been seen with the introduction of optical coherence interferometry and immersion ultrasonography, but in order to optimize their use it is essential that biometrists are able to assess the resultant scans correctly. If all the factors outlined throughout this chapter are considered, the likelihood of achieving post-operative refractive success and patient satisfaction will be significantly increased.

Acknowledgements

I would like to thank both David Sculfor, head optometrist at Stoke Mandeville Hospital, and Lyn Millbank, orthoptist and clinical trainer, for all their assistance and guidance.

Further reading

Barnard, N.A.S. (2004). *Assessment of the Anterior Chamber: Tutorials*. American Academy of Optometry, British Chapter.

doctor-hill.com website: www.doctor-hill.com/physicians/physician_main.htm.

Haigis W., Lege B., Miller N. and Schneider B. (2000). Comparison of immersion ultrasound biometry and partial coherence interferometry for intraocular lens calculation according to Haigis. *Graefe's Arch. Clin. Exp. Ophthalmol.* **238**: 765–773.

Holladay J.T. (1989). IOL calculations following RK. *Refract. Corneal Surg.* **5**: 203.

Kim, Y.L., Walsh, J.T., Goldstick, T.K. and Glucksberg, M.R. (2004). Variation of corneal refractive index with hydration. *Phys. Med. Biol.* **49**: 859–868.

Langenbucher, A., Haigis, W., Seitz, B. (2004). Difficult lens power calculations. *Curr. Opin. Ophthalmol.* **15**(11): 1–9.

Nemeth, J., Fekete, O. and Pesztenlehrer, N. (2003). Optical and ultrasound measurement of axial length and anterior chamber depth for intraocular lens power calculation. *J. Cat. Ref. Surg.* **29**(1): 85–88.

Roberts D. (1996). *Ocular Disease and Treatment*, 2nd edition. Butterworth-Heinemann: 293–311.

Royal College of Ophthalmologists website: www.rcophth.ac.uk/scientific/publications

Schachar, R.A, Levy, N.S. and Bonney, A.C. (1980). Accuracy of intraocular lens powers calculated from A Scan biometry with the Echo-Oculometer. *Ophthalmic Surg.* **11**: 865–858.

Shammas, H.J., Shammas, M.C., Garabet, A., Kim, J.H., Shammas, A. and LaBree, L. (2003). Correcting the corneal power measurements for intraocular lens power calculations after myopic laser *in situ* keratomileusis. *Am. J. Ophthalmol.* **136**(3): 426–432.

ULIB website: www.augenklinik.uni-wuerzburg.de/eulib/const.htm

Waldron, R.G. A-scan biometry pages: emedicine.com/oph/topic486.htm

4

Recent advances in intraocular lens technology

Richard Packard

Introduction

Since 1949, when Harold Ridley began the era of modern cataract surgery, there has been continual evolution to try to emulate the visual range of the young phakic adult. The first stage was to establish the efficacy of intraocular lens (IOL) implantation. When ultrasonic biometry became standard in the early 1980s the range of lens powers increased enormously as cataract surgery started to become a refractive procedure. However, although excellent visual results for best corrected distance vision could now be achieved, it was not until foldable IOLs became generally available, with further reduction of incision size due to phacoemulsification, that unaided vision caught up. Although patients were very happy to be able to see in the distance without glasses, the majority still needed reading glasses most of the time. In order to try and deal with this pseudophakic presbyopia, and thus make patients spectacle independent, IOL manufacturers needed to devise means to allow good reading as well. This has led to a variety of approaches based on different technologies, some of which have worked better than others. None is yet as good as the visual capabilities of a 20-year-old emmetrope. Despite this, however, results are now good enough in refractive terms that the removal of lenses from presbyopes without cataract will become increasingly common.

For those patients who do not wish to go down the multifocal route there are also new types of monofocal lenses to enhance the visual result further. These include IOLs with aspheric optics to improve contrast sensitivity in mesopic and scotopic conditions, toric lenses to correct pre-existing corneal astigmatism and lenses with tints to block potentially damaging wavelengths of visible light. In the near future all of these different improvements will be incorporated in multifocal lenses as required.

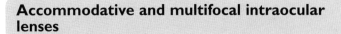

Accommodative and multifocal intraocular lenses

Available technologies

Two very different approaches have been tried to date: accommodative lenses and pseudoaccommodative lenses.

Accommodative lenses

The first type of accommodative IOLs work on the principle of movement of the pseudophakos in the eye. This is supposed to happen under the influence of the vitreous pressure changing during accommodative effort; a 1 mm movement forward producing 1.5 D of change in the lens power. The two main lenses that have been investigated in this regard and brought to market are the Crystalens from Eyeonics (Figure 4.1) and the Human Optics 1CU (Figure 4.2). Although the results published for both lenses initially looked promising they have largely been unsustained. This is due to changes in the capsular bag over time and much less movement than predicted for the lens. There were also issues due to high rates of posterior capsular opacification. These two lenses will have limited appeal in the future, although FDA studies with the Crystalens have shown very good intermediate vision for a high proportion of patients.

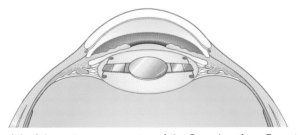

Figure 4.1   Schematic representation of the Crystalens from Eyeonics

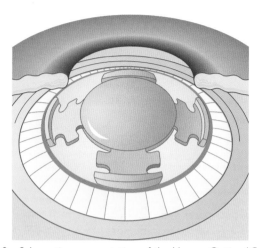

Figure 4.2 Schematic representation of the Human Optics 1CU

In order to increase the accommodative effect, a lens has been designed (Visiogen Synchrony lens) that incorporates two optics in the capsular bag. Here the small movements which are achievable due to vitreous pressure are considerably enhanced, with 4 to 6 D of accommodation on offer. The problem with lenses of this type is that they tend to hold the capsular bag open, allowing development of Elschnig pearls and thus visual loss until a capsulotomy has been performed. Various novel devices are currently under review to try to address this issue. One of these is the Perfect Capsule, where the capsular bag is sealed and irrigated with deionized water to cause epithelial cells within the capsular bag to hydrolyse.

There have also been a number of attempts to devise a phakoersatz, by refilling the emptied capsular bag with some substance that will be able to act under the influence of the ciliary muscles to change shape and thus accommodate. This may ultimately prove the most fruitful of all. Perhaps the most exciting development is the *NuLens* accommodating IOL. It is unique in that it is designed to change its true power during accommodation and it has been shown in an animal model to deliver more than 40 D of accommodation. The *NuLens* is the

brainchild of Dr Joshua Ben-Nun of Israel. It incorporates a small
chamber of silicone gel and a posterior piston with an aperture in
its centre that allows the gel to bulge relative to the forces
generated by accommodation. The lens is fixated in the sulcus
without sutures in front of the collapsed capsular bag, zonules
and ciliary processes. Initial human studies have shown 8 D of
accommodation.

Pseudoaccommodative lenses

Diffractive lenses
In 1989 the 3M company introduced a rigid diffractive multifocal
made of polymethyl methacrylate (PMMA). For some patients this
lens worked very well as the reading addition was the equivalent
of 3 D at the spectacle plane. However the lens had a variety of
drawbacks. First, as it was PMMA it was rigid and thus required
an incision of 6 to 7 mm. This of itself was not so much of an
issue, but many of the investigators were still using large incision
extracapsular techniques, which made control of post-operative
astigmatism a potential problem. With pseudoaccommodative
lenses, more than 1 D of astigmatism considerably diminishes the
unaided function of the lens. Also, because of the light distribution
between near and far with this lens, night vision was
compromised. However the lens showed what might be possible
with improvements in design and foldable lens materials.

It is helpful to review here what diffraction is and why it can be
used for lenses of this type to extend the range of a patient's vision.
Diffraction is the bending of light around edges or corners. It can be
harnessed to control and focus light; this is achieved by altering the
shape and spacing of steps known as gratings (Figure 4.3). By varying
the line spacing of a diffraction grating it is possible to alter the angle
of diffraction and thus to create more than one focal point. If the
height of the steps on a diffraction grating is changed the amount of
energy directed to each focal point generated can be set; this is
dependent on the fact that light travels in waves. In order to put a
diffraction grating on to a surface, concentric rings are created.

On the 3M lens and most diffractive IOLs the light is split
equally between near and far. In practice it is not possible with

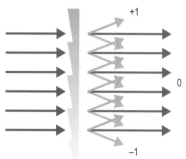

- Triangular steps of transparent material

- Light diffracts from the steps and is primarily split into three beams

- Angle of steps shifts the amount of energy in each order

Figure 4.3 Diffraction grating

full optic diffractive lenses to use more than 80% of the available light. Thus with half this going to near and half to distance only 40% will be available for each. This explains why mesopic and scotopic vision is compromised with lenses of this type. Various methods are being tried to overcome this problem. On two of the full optic diffractive IOLs (AMO Tecnis MF and AcriTec) some form of asphericity is used to enhance contrast sensitivity in low light. Although this improves things the full aperture lenses of this type still have problems with haloes at night.

There is an alternative approach, where both refractive and diffractive elements in the lens are important. The Alcon ReStor (Figure 4.4) has a central diffraction grating of 3.6 mm in diameter. The grating is apodized, which means that there is a gradual modification in the optical properties of a lens from its centre to its edge. This is used to reduce the effects of diffraction

Figure 4.4 Alcon ReStor lens

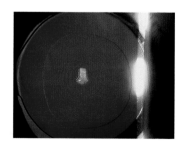

in the lens periphery. Apodization is routinely used in microscopy and astronomy to reduce diffractive halos. In the ReStor lens the step heights vary from 1.3 μm centrally to 0.4 μm peripherally. The spacings between the steps also decrease towards the periphery. Outside the diffractive zone the lens is refractive; this means that as the pupil dilates in low light the light split goes from near to distance (see Figure 4.5). Thus with a 2 mm pupil 60% of available light goes to distance and 40% to near. When the pupil dilates to 6 mm the split is 90% distance and 10% near. This change also considerably reduces haloes around lights at night. All diffractive multifocals give excellent near vision, with 3.5 to 4 D incorporated at the lens plane and between 2.75 and 3.2 D at the spectacle plane.

Refractive lenses
The other main group of pseudoaccommodative IOLs is those using refractive technology. Refraction is the bending of waves that occurs when a wavefront passes obliquely from one medium to another. The phenomenon is most familiar with light waves.

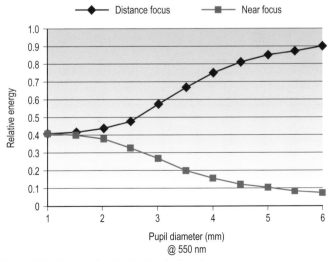

Figure 4.5 Energy distribution for ReStor lens

When light passes from a less dense medium (for example, aqueous) to a more dense one (for example, an IOL), it is refracted towards the normal (an imaginary line perpendicular to the surface). This occurs because the light waves are slowed down by the denser medium, causing them to change direction. The opposite effect occurs as the wavefront passes out the other side of the lens. The curvature of the IOL will modify the direction the light wave takes as it passes on.

There have been a number of different types of refractive IOLs. The early designs from IoLab and Storz were near-dominant with a central reading add. Patients read well, but if their pupils constricted too much in bright light their distance vision was compromised. These designs have long since been abandoned.

The first multifocal to be used in large numbers was the Array lens made by AMO (Figure 4.6). It is a zonal refractive lens; it has a central distance zone surrounded by a near zone, then another distance zone and another near zone, and finally another distance zone outside of that. The reading add equates to about 2.25 D at the spectacle plane. Patients usually have good distance vision but

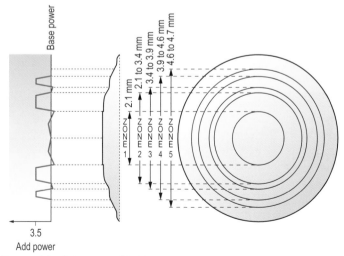

Figure 4.6 Schematic of AMO Array lens

reading in bright light can be pupil dependent. The concentric nature of the zones on lens optic means that all patients have some halo effect at night. Most get used to it, however, after a few months. In the latest version of this type of lens from AMO, called the ReZoom, the light distribution has been altered between the zones and the blending is better. The reading add is stronger and overall the patient satisfaction seems to be higher. (Outcomes are discussed later in this chapter). The Rayner company has just started investigations with their M-flex, a new refractive IOL based on its C-flex platform. Little information is currently available about this lens.

As already mentioned, in order for multifocal IOLs to function properly it is necessary to reduce any pre-existing corneal astigmatism to less than 1 D. There are various ways of doing this, depending on the amount of reduction required. The simplest, if there is 1.5 D or less, is to operate on the steep corneal axis, possibly enlarging the wound to 3.5 mm. For amounts up to 2.5 D, limbal relaxing incisions (LRIs) work well when the incisions are of the correct depth and the nomogram is used correctly. LRIs are probably the most popular technique at present. It is possible to use the excimer laser to correct this astigmatism and any residual refractive error. However this is another procedure, and many would prefer to complete the surgery all at once. Finally, as mentioned above, toric multifocals should be available soon and simplify this problem.

Pros and cons of different multifocal lens styles

It is clear that there are many options out there for patients. How do we decide which multifocal lens to use, or whether to use one at all? The patient's perception of what he or she wants to achieve visually after the surgery and their occupational considerations will have great influence. For example, a diffractive lens works well for people who read a lot, although the reading distance will almost certainly diminish. However a full aperture diffractive lens will cause more visual disturbance with lights at night. The ReStor may be the choice here because of its combined diffractive approach. For patients who spend considerable time in front of a computer, intermediate vision is most important. Diffractive IOLs tend not to have such good intermediate vision, so a lens like the ReZoom or the Crystalens may work better here, with the proviso that reading glasses might be needed more often. If night driving is an important part of a patient's life, most multifocals may cause some initial difficulties with haloes at night. Although this undoubtedly gets better with time, refractive and full aperture diffractives do least well here. Again the ReStor may be the best compromise, or a monofocal may be appropriate if the patient is concerned about this. A discussion of these sort of issues forms part of the informed consent prior to surgery, partly to establish information about lifestyle but more importantly to avoid unrealistic expectations.

Patients to avoid as candidates for multifocal implantation

Most patients can, with appropriate counselling, be candidates for implantation of multifocal lenses. In practice, however, in the UK because of cost considerations these lenses will probably be mainly used in the private sector for both cataract and refractive lens exchange (RLE) patients. There are, however, certain groups to treat with caution:

- Those with unrealistic expectations of what can be achieved and who do not listen to advice.
- Low myopes who currently read well without glasses, even if they have cataract. Even though the reading may be very good with lenses such as the ReStor or Tecnis MF, it will not be as good as that with the patients' own eyes. These patients will probably be happiest continuing to use distance-only glasses after surgery.
- Patients with advanced glaucomatous visual loss. Their contrast sensitivity is already compromised; losing even a little bit more from use of multifocal IOLs is probably ill advised.
- Patients with age-related or diabetic maculopathy will not do well.
- Occupational night drivers, although this is a relative contraindication.

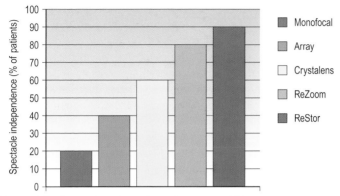

Figure 4.7 Spectacle independence for various IOLs

Visual results after implantation

What sort of visual results can patients expect after implantation
with modern multifocal IOLs? Since spectacle independence is the
end result that patients are seeking, this will give us an indication
(Figure 4.7). In the author's own series of over 200 patients
implanted bilaterally with the ReStor lens, 92% do not use glasses
at all and none of the remainder wear glasses all of the time.
Most of those using glasses occasionally do this for intermediate
tasks, such as computer use. As far as unwanted visual
phenomena are concerned, such as haloes at night, the
percentage who notice this is 10%, of whom three patients are at
all bothered. These patients are still delighted to have had the
ReStor lens at their surgery as their vision is so good in all other
respects. All of the above needs to be considered when talking to
patients about lenses of this type.

Aspheric intraocular lenses

Spherical aberration is a function of most IOLs because they are
biconvex. The further from the centre of the lens the light is
refracted, the more the focal point moves from that of the light

passing through near the centre. In practice this does not matter with pupil sizes of 4 mm or less, but once the pupil size enlarges beyond this, as in low light, this slight blurring of the image causes loss of contrast sensitivity. In the young eye the cornea is negatively prolate; this is counteracted by the positive prolateness of the lens. As the lens ages it becomes more negatively prolate and so spherical aberration does increase, but of course not as much as when the lens is removed.

It may be helpful to define here the term prolate. Prolate is the shape of a spheroid (which is a three-dimensional surface obtained by rotating an ellipse about one of its principal axes) where the ellipse is rotated about its major axis. If the minor axis is chosen, the surface is called an oblate spheroid. The cornea is qualitatively prolate or oblate, depending on whether it is stretched or flattened in its axial dimension. In a prolate cornea the meridional curvature decreases from pole to equator, and in an oblate cornea the meridional curvature continually increases.

The optical surfaces of the normal human eye, both cornea and lens, are prolate. This shape has an optical advantage because it tends to compensate spherical aberration. Changes in the spherical aberration of the crystalline lens have been implicated with this type of vision decline. Between the ages of 20 and 70 years, total wavefront aberration of the eye increases more than 300%. Total aberrations in young people are low because the optical characteristics of the young crystalline lens compensate for the aberrations in the cornea. As a person ages, his or her lenses do not compensate as well because the magnitude and the sign of the spherical aberration of the lenses changes significantly, leading to degradation of optical quality.

The first IOL that attempted to correct this was the AMO Tecnis Z9000 lens. It was designed with an aspheric front surface that had been chosen by using information from wavefront scans of the eye. Contrast sensitivity studies showed a distinct improvement in performance at low light levels. This has prompted other manufacturers of IOLs to produce aspheric lenses. Alcon has the IQ lens, where the posterior surface has been made aspheric; this has enabled the lens overall to be 9% thinner (Figure 4.8), which will also aid implantation through a

AcrySof IQ IOL

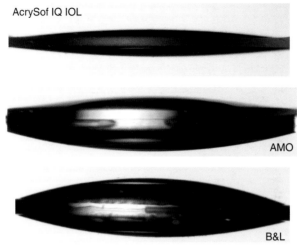

AMO

B&L

Actual digital photos of 20D lens comparisons

Figure 4.8 Profiles of aspheric IOLs

smaller incision. Bausch and Lomb has the AO lens, and AcriTec and Rayner are also moving into this field. This type of lens will become the standard approach over the next few years. Although not all the lenses of this type are of similar efficiency they are at least a big improvement on biconvex lenses. Figure 4.9 shows the modulation transfer function (MTF), a laboratory measure of the optical quality of a lens, of three different IOLs. It seems surprising, considering how long spectacle and camera lenses have been aspheric, that IOL manufacturers have taken so long to develop aspheric IOLs.

Toric lenses

As already mentioned, it is now possible to use an IOL to correct corneal astigmatism rather than having to correct the shape of the cornea. There have been a number of different designs of

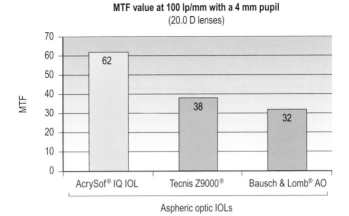

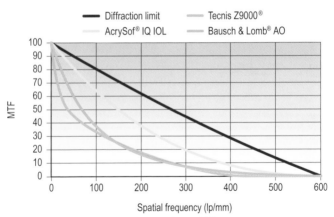

Figure 4.9 TF values for various aspheric IOLs

toric IOL, but whichever one is used it is essential that the lens does not rotate once lined up on the mark placed on the outside of the eye before surgery. A shift of 10 degrees results in loss of one-third of the astigmatic correction; 30 degrees of movement and you might as well not have implanted a toric lens as no correction will remain. Staar produced the first foldable toric IOL, however this silicone plate haptic lens was not stable enough in the capsular bag. Both Rayner and Alcon have toric lenses; Rayner's is on its C-flex platform, and Alcon's is based on its SN60 single-piece lens. Both of the generic platforms have been shown to be very stable within the capsular bag and results for both of these toric lenses are very promising.

Lenses with filters

IOLs have included filters for ultraviolet light since the mid 1980s because it was felt to be retinotoxic. A number of studies, both laboratory and epidemiological, have suggested that some wavelengths in the blue/violet part of the visible spectrum may be damaging to the retina. Two manufacturers (Hoya and Alcon) (Figure 4.10) currently have lenses that filter this part of the spectrum. There is considerable debate within the ophthalmic community as to the merits of this type of filtering; there is feeling that the evidence for retinal damage is too circumstantial and that such filtering interferes with scotopic vision and colour vision. There is, however, little evidence to support this view. In fact increasing numbers of lens manufacturers are considering

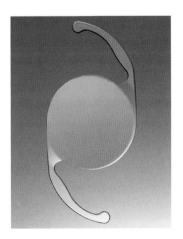

Figure 4.10   Acrysof natural IOL

some form of filtering, albeit of a slightly reduced range of wavelengths. Patients' own natural lenses provide this filtering prior to removal, and so as refractive lens exchange becomes a more common event such filtering will be considered mandatory.

Further reading

Ophthalmic Hyperguide website: www.ophthalmic.hyperguides.com

5
Techniques in cataract surgery

Raman Malhotra

History of cataract surgery

In ancient times, cataract was not recognized as opacification of the crystalline lens, rather it was thought to be a suffusion forming between the pupil and the lens. The term cataract therefore arose after translation of the Arabic term for 'suffusion' into the Latin *cataracta* (meaning waterfall or obstruction of flow), similar to the cataracts that impeded the navigation of the Nile river.

Couching

Surgical treatment of cataracts began with couching, described in India by Sushruta as early 800 BC. A needle was passed through the sclera or cornea to push the white lens downward or backwards into the vitreous cavity. Patients were able to see forms and figures afterwards. In the middle ages, couchers travelled from town to town and using a common sewing needle would couch cataracts in the village square. Complication rates were obviously high, and a couching procedure was considered a success if the patient was able to ambulate without assistance.

Extracapsular cataract extraction

Cataract surgery then advanced to extracapsular cataract extraction (ECCE): the extraction rather than simple displacement of the cataract (Jacques Daviel 1696–1762, Albrecht von Graefe 1828–1870). The procedure was performed most safely after the cortex had liquefied, therefore surgery was delayed until the cataract was 'ripe'. This technique did not gain wide acceptance due to the significant risks of endophthalmitis, incomplete cortex removal, chronic inflammation, capsular opacification and pupil block glaucoma.

Intracapsular cataract extraction

Due to the problems of extracapsular extraction, the technique evolved to the removal of the entire lens from the eye. Lysis of the zonular fibres was a problem, but the use of the cryoprobe in 1961, and subsequently chemical disillusion with the enzyme alpha-chymotrypsin, improved the safety of intracapsular extraction to make it a very successful procedure. Published results showed 85% of patients achieving a best corrected visual acuity of 6/9 or better. Over 5% of patients, however, were rendered blind due to complications, such as infection, haemorrhage, retinal detachment or cystoid macular oedema. Furthermore these patients required aphakic spectacles, with their inherent problems.

Modern extracapsular cataract extraction

By preserving the posterior lens capsule, the risk of vitreous loss, and therefore many of the potentially blinding complications, may be reduced. With the growing use of the operating microscope, this technique evolved alongside better ways of removing residual cortical material. This technique continued to be the procedure of choice during the 1980s and early 1990s.

Sutureless extracapsular cataract extraction

Despite all the modern advances in cataract surgery, the greatest challenge continues to be the large amount of cataract blindness in developing countries. Millions of people in the developing nations with reversible blindness due to cataracts continue to go untreated, and modern phacoemulsification technology is too expensive to purchase and maintain in these areas. Furthermore, the more advanced cataracts seen in these populations make phacoemulsification difficult and expensive and lead to a higher risk of complications.

For these patients, a high-volume, low-cost, low-technology procedure that can deal with advanced cataracts but which avoids the problems related to sutures and has a low complication rate is the paradigm.

Small incision or sutureless extracapsular cataract extraction (SECCE) has emerged as the procedure of choice for the developing world. The entire nucleus followed by cortex is

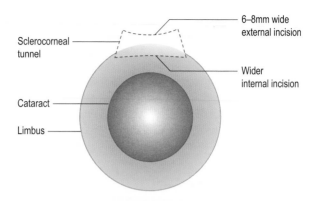

Sclerocorneal tunnel

6–8mm wide external incision

Wider internal incision

Cataract

Limbus

Figure 5.1 Sutureless extracapsular cataract extraction (SECCE) through a 6–8 mm self-sealing sclerocorneal tunnel

removed through a 6–8 mm self-sealing sclerocorneal tunnel (Figure 5.1) and a single-piece rigid polymethyl methacrylate (PMMA) posterior chamber intraocular lens (IOL) implant is then inserted into the capsular bag.

By alternating between two parallel operating tables a single surgeon is able to perform over 15 cases per hour (Figure 5.2). Despite the high proportion of advanced and mature cataracts, the operative complication rate is low, with vitreous loss occurring in fewer than 1% of cases. Visual outcomes are also excellent, with approximately 80% of patients seeing 6/18 or better uncorrected in contrast to 90% of these patients seeing 6/60 or worse pre-operatively.

Phacoemulsification cataract surgery

The principles of modern cataract surgery are based on phacoemulsification cataract extraction through small incisions. Foldable IOL implants are standard and virtually all surgery is

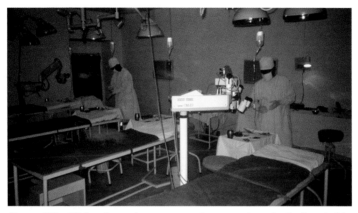

Figure 5.2 High-volume daycase operating room in a charity hospital in Rajasthan, India. A microscope revolves between two parallel operating tables to allow a single surgeon to perform up to 15 cases an hour

now carried out under local anaesthesia, the majority being topical anaesthesia and as a daycase procedure.

Daycase surgery

For routine, uncomplicated cataract surgery, discharge on the same day is now the norm. Adequate provision of transport is required, along with a friend or relative to escort the patient on the day of surgery. Patients who live on their own usually do not require to be accompanied overnight.

Local anaesthesia

Over 90% of cataract operations in the UK are performed under local anaesthesia. The two most popular methods are sub-Tenon's anaesthesia and topical anaesthesia. Sub-Tenon's anaesthesia is delivered using a blunt-tipped cannula directly to the sub-Tenon's space following dissection through the conjunctiva and Tenon's capsule in the region of the inferonasal conjunctival fornix (Figure 5.3). This provides excellent retrobulbar anaesthesia and

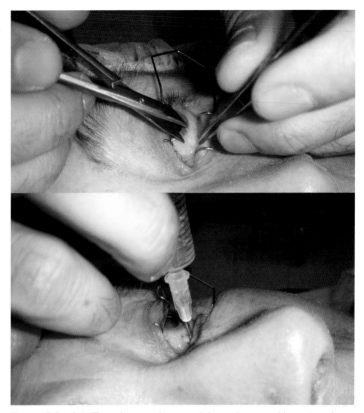

Figure 5.3 Sub-Tenon's anaesthesia is delivered using a blunt-tipped cannula directly to the sub-Tenon's space following dissection through the conjunctiva and Tenon's capsule in the region of the inferonasal conjunctival fornix

minimizes the risk of a penetrating globe injury (a well known risk following traditional peribulbar or retrobulbar injections). Patient satisfaction is high using this technique, even compared with topical anaesthesia. Topical anaesthesia, by way of drops only to anaesthetize the eye, is administered before surgery. It can be complemented by intravenous sedation and also by intracameral anaesthesia by way of unpreserved local anaesthetic injection into the anterior chamber at the time of surgery, if required. It is observed that without intracameral anaesthesia, although surgery is surprisingly pain free, patients often experience an ache at times, particularly if a change in anterior chamber depth occurs suddenly during surgery.

Small incision

Incision size in cataract surgery continues to reduce through developments in surgical technology, both of phacoemulsification and of lens implant design. Incisions no longer require to be sutured, are now typically 3 mm in size and are self-sealing by way of a two-plane construction and internal tamponade by intraocular fluid pressure. Small incision surgery has also resulted in a decline in wound rupture following blunt injury, as typically seen in ECCE wounds. Furthermore, based on studies examining the pressure required to rupture a cadaveric globe, it is remarkable that the eye will rupture at its weakest point, namely the insertion of the recti, rather than at the site of the phaco wound.

Small incisions are considered to be astigmatically neutral and contribute to rapid visual rehabilitation following surgery. In addition, the need to avoid bending or straining following small incision cataract surgery is less essential.

Site of incision

Small incisions for phacoemulsification cataract surgery may be clear corneal (at the corneal limbus, Figure 5.4) or sclerocorneal (a scleral tunnel is constructed, beginning 2 mm posterior to the limbus and entering the anterior chamber approximately 1.5 mm anterior to the limbus).

It is believed that scleral tunnel incisions induce less astigmatic change in comparison with clear corneal incisions. However, the potential for wound-related complications is a little greater for sclerocorneal incisions, in particular hyphaema, delayed filtering blebs and early discomfort.

Figure 5.4 Corneal limbal tunnel incision

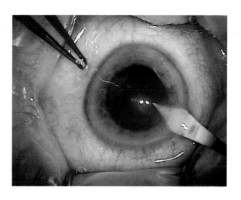

The site of incision also varies, either being placed between the superior limbus or temporally. Temporal incisions are often used to overcome a prominent brow, however there are other advantages. The temporal site is furthest from the visual axis, therefore providing more space to manoeuvre during surgery. As corneal incisions tend to relax the corneal curvature along that particular meridian, temporal incisions help in facilitating post-operative 'with-the-rule' astigmatism following surgery, an advantage for elderly patients. To this purpose, many surgeons routinely aim to place incisions 'on-axis', along the steepest meridian.

Corneal sutures

Placement of sutures is nowadays a rare occurrence during routine phacoemulsification cataract surgery. Sutures are indicated if the incision is unlikely to seal completely, thereby increasing the risks of aqueous leak and hypotony or of tear flow into the anterior chamber and possible microbial contamination. Such a scenario may arise if the tunnel is of inadequate length or is too wide (usually greater than 4 mm). A corneal burn may also cause sufficient contraction to prevent self-sealing and require suture placement. Other indications for suture placement include persistent iris prolapse and poor patient compliance (and risk of self-injury post-operatively), and sutures may be required following complicated cataract surgery, for example vitreous loss.

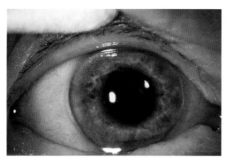

Figure 5.5   A corneal suture placed at the end of cataract surgery. The knot should be buried within the corneal stroma so as not to cause ocular discomfort and a foreign-body sensation to the patient

Nylon sutures are used due to their strength, elasticity, monofilament properties and slow reabsorption with minimal inflammation (Figure 5.5). Sutures are generally removed at 6 weeks post-operatively. They may, however, be allowed to remain, for example if concern exists over the integrity of the wound, or where removal may result in an undesirable change in refractive astigmatism. Nylon sutures gradually dissolve over 18 months and patients remain asymptomatic.

Viscoelastic

The development of viscoelastic technology stands alongside the introduction of the operating microscope in improving the safety and results of modern cataract surgery. A viscous clear biocompatible gel, for example sodium hyaluronate, is used to inflate the anterior chamber to allow capsulorrhexis. Viscoelastic is also injected following lens removal into the anterior chamber and the capsular bag to allow safe IOL implantation. Viscoelastic materials possess a unique ability, based on their chemical structure, to protect the corneal endothelium from mechanical trauma, and they maintain an intraocular space in the anterior chamber. They can also be used to manipulate intraocular structures directly while preventing mechanical damage to tissue and avoiding adhesions post-operatively. Substances currently used include sodium hyaluronate (Healon), chondroitin sulphate (Viscoat) and hydroxypropyl methylcellulose (HPMC).

The main disadvantage of using viscoelastic is the significant elevation of intraocular pressure seen post-operatively if any is retained (not completely removed during surgery). It is presumed that this is the result of large molecules of viscoelastic creating mechanical resistance in the trabecular meshwork. The pressure spike typically resolves within 72 hours.

Capsulorrhexis

During traditional ECCE the anterior capsule was opened by using a series of stab incisions lined in a circular manner to form a large 'can-opener' capsulotomy. However, due to the increased manipulation of the nucleus within the capsule during phacoemulsification, any point of weakness in the capsulotomy would easily result in a radial tear, which may extend to the equator or even beyond to involve the posterior capsule.

In the mid 1980s a continuous circular capsular tear, known as the capsulorrhexis, was developed so that no point of weakness would exist in the anterior capsular opening. The stress distribution at the edge of the capsulorrhexis is uniform and therefore low at any point, thereby providing a strong capsulorrhexis edge that is resistant to tearing (Figure 5.6).

Figure 5.6 Capsulorrhexis: (a) being carried out, and (b) the clear edge of the capsulorrhexis following removal of the lens. The cannula is injecting viscoelastic into the capsular bag

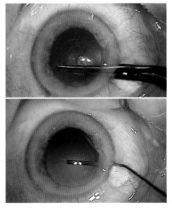

a

b

Hydrodissection

Following capsulorrhexis, a gentle injection of balanced saline solution (fluid with physiological pH, osmolarity and mineral content) is placed between the lens capsule and cortex to separate the lens from the capsule and mobilize the lens prior to phacoemulsification. A typical wave of fluid is seen passing behind and across the lens within the view of the operating microscope, confirming that this has been completed (Figure 5.7).

Phacoemulsification

In 1967 Kelman described a single-instrument technique for cataract removal using ultrasound. The technique employs an ultrasound probe, which uses a piezoelectric crystal to convert electrical energy into vibrating shockwave energy. In a manner similar to a hammer drill, the vibrations are used to liquefy the hard nucleus.

There are a number of phacoemulsification techniques used to break the lens up within the capsular bag. Divide and conquer and phaco-chop are among the most popular techniques currently used. The term 'divide and conquer' was coined to describe techniques whereby the nucleus is systematically divided and then fragmented, rather than randomly emulsified (Figure 5.8). The phaco-chop technique, introduced by Nagahara in 1993, uses the principle of splitting wood to fracture the nucleus; a chopping

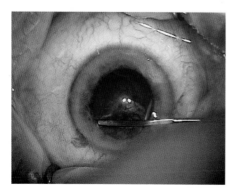

Figure 5.7
Hydrodissection: a hydrodissection cannula allows gentle injection of saline solution between the lens capsule and cortex. The typical wave of fluid is seen passing across and behind the lens

Figure 5.8 Divide and conquer technique: systematic division and fragmentation of the nucleus

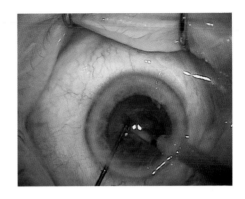

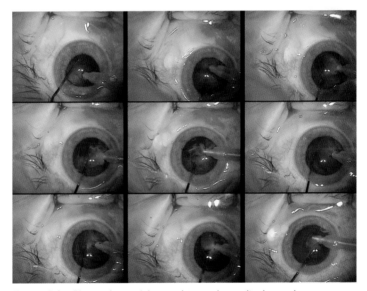

Figure 5.9 Phaco-chop: a 'chopper' is used to split the nucleus once impaled by the phacoemulsification tip

instrument is used to split the nucleus once it is impaled by the phacoemulsification tip (Figure 5.9). The main advantage of the phaco-chop technique is that it minimizes the amount of phacoemulsification time and energy used, thereby minimizing corneal endothelium loss. A disadvantage to the technique is the greater care that is required to prevent anterior capsule tear when inserting the chopper at the edge of the nucleus.

Laser cataract surgery

It is a common misperception among patients that cataract surgery is performed using a laser. Use of lasers such as the erbium:YAG laser has, however, shown promise as a new emerging technique for lens nucleus removal. Studies have shown that the laser energy dissipated by an internal probe is localized and with possibly less heat emission in comparison with traditional ultrasonic phacoemulsification techniques. There also seems to be very little difference in outcomes when compared with conventional surgery techniques. However, laser is considered less effective, particularly when dealing with dense cataracts, and does not have any obvious benefit with regards to reducing corneal endothelial loss. The main use for laser in cataract surgery therefore remains for posterior capsulotomy as a treatment for post-operative posterior capsule opacification.

Microincision phacoemulsification cataract surgery

Corneal incision size continues to decrease such that an emerging technique known as bimanual phacoemulsification has emerged. Surgery is performed through incisions less than 2 mm in size. The main purpose for reducing the incision size is to reduce surgically induced astigmatism and wound-related complications. The traditional coaxial phacoemulsification probe is split so that the irrigation and aspiration components are separated and are carried out through two microincisions. The theoretical benefits of separating these components through two microincisions are to stabilize the anterior chamber and to improve fluidics during surgery. This may be of particular benefit in young patients, in whom a stable anterior chamber may minimize shifts of the vitreous and therefore help reduce the risk of retinal tears. Although outcomes of microincision bimanual surgery have been reported, studies comparing microincision and coaxial phacoemulsification suggest that total phacoemulsification time can be further lowered and that surgically induced astigmatism can be reduced using bimanual techniques. However, at present, the wound then needs to be enlarged in order to insert any of the currently available IOL implants. The next step is therefore to develop injectable IOL implants that can be inserted through smaller incisions than currently possible.

Intraocular lens implantation

Rigid PMMA IOLs have now been largely superseded by foldable IOLs made of silicone, acrylics or hydrogels. Foldable IOLs allow 6 mm diameter optics to be inserted through 3.2 mm incisions (Figure 5.10 and Figure 5.11). These can also be injected by way

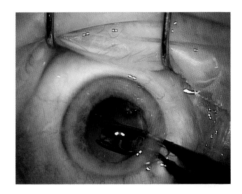

Figure 5.10
Insertion of a folded acrylic IOL implant

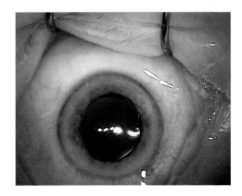

Figure 5.11 Folded acrylic IOL implant following insertion into the capsular bag

of injectable devices. IOL implants are discussed in detail in Chapter 4.

Complications during cataract surgery

Operative complications are an inevitable risk during cataract surgery and can occur at any stage during surgery. Each step during phacoemulsification relies on the success of the previous one. A poorly constructed wound could leak during surgery, resulting in an unstable anterior chamber and an endothelial, iris or capsular injury. If the capsulorrhexis is too small, it may be damaged by the phaco probe. The tear may extend into the posterior capsule, resulting in vitreous loss. Any error at any stage during surgery can have a cascading effect, magnifying the damage.

Significant and well-recognized intraoperative complications are detailed below.

Complications during regional anaesthesia

Retrobulbar or intraorbital haemorrhage is a rare, sight-threatening complication that may occur immediately following retrobulbar or peribulbar anaesthesia. It is immediately recognized as acute proptosis, tenseness of the orbital contents and difficulty separating the eyelids. This may require an emergency lateral canthomy to release any orbital tightening and usually results in postponement of surgery.

Globe perforation as a complication of retrobulbar or peribulbar anaesthesia is well documented. This is due to the use of a needle and may not be recognized at the time of administering anaesthesia. Such a complication may only be identified post-operatively if vision remains poor due to vitreous haemorrhage or an early retinal detachment. Eyes with staphylomata, or thin sclera due to high myopia, may be at particular risk.

Regional anaesthesia, including sub-Tenon's, carries the risk of prolonged strabismus and diplopia. Vertical diplopia due to restriction of the inferior rectus muscle is thought to occur in approximately 0.5% of cataract procedures and may require subsequent squint surgery.

Conjunctival inclusion cysts are also known to occur at any conjunctival entry site.

Corneal complications during surgery

A tear in Descemet's membrane usually occurs if a blunt instrument has been inserted or when fluid is inadvertently injected between Descemet's membrane and the corneal stroma. It results in corneal stromal swelling and epithelial bullae in a localized area of the detachment, usually near the incision site. Small detachments may resolve spontaneously or they may be reattached with an injection of air into the anterior chamber for tamponade. Large detachments rarely need suturing into place.

Corneal thermal burns may occur at the tunnel due to transfer of heat from the phaco probe, particularly if the wound is too tight or the probe is pressed against the corneal lip, thereby preventing adequate flow of irrigation along the probe. This can produce clouding of the cornea and contraction at this site and may result in wound leak as well as significant astigmatism post-operatively.

Capsule rupture during surgery

This serious complication, and one of the most significant, is estimated to occur in 1% of phacoemulsification cataract procedures. It can occur at any one of four main stages during cataract surgery:

- at the time of hydrodissection
- during phacoemulsification
- during removal of cortex
- during insertion of the IOL.

The principles of dealing with this complication include:

1. safe removal of the remaining lens material
2. an anterior vitrectomy to remove vitreous carefully from the anterior chamber and the incision sites, and

3. preservation of remaining capsule in order to allow support for a posterior chamber IOL.

The visual results after capsule rupture are not as good as after uncomplicated surgery. Studies suggest that approximately 85% of patients subsequently achieve vision of 6/12 or better. Poor vision in the remaining 15% is often due to cystoid macular oedema.

Choroidal haemorrhage or effusion

Choroidal haemorrhage or effusion occurs in approximately 0.1% of cases and causes a forward shift of the iris–lens diaphragm, with prolapse of posterior structures and a change in the red reflex. Effusion may be a precursor to haemorrhage, although it may be difficult to differentiate the two. It is uncertain why this complication occurs but it is presumably due to leakage or rupture of choroidal vasculature, and it is considered to occur more often in patients with underlying systemic vascular disease, hypertension, obesity, glaucoma or chronic ocular inflammation.

Rapid wound closure is required once this complication is recognized in order to prevent iris prolapse and expulsion of the lens, vitreous and blood (expulsive choroidal haemorrhage). Sclerostomies may also be performed using a blade or small trephine to drain blood posterior to the ora serrata.

Further reading

Burrato, L., Werner, L., Zanini, M. and Apple, D.J. (2003). *Phacoemulsification: Principles and Techniques*, 2nd edition. Slack Inc.

Chang, D.F. (2005). Tackling the greatest challenge in cataract surgery. *Br. J. Ophthalmol.* **89**: 1073–1077.

Hennig, A., Kumar, J., Yorston, D. and Foster, A. (2003). Sutureless cataract surgery with nucleus extraction: outcome of a prospective study in Nepal. *Br. J. Ophthalmol.* **87**: 266–270.

Paul, T. and Braga-Mele, R. (2005). Bimanual microincisional phacoemulsification: the future of cataract surgery? *Curr. Opin. Ophthalmol.* **16**(1): 2–7.

Rosenfeld, S.I. (2006). Basic and Clinical Science Course Section 11: Lens and cataract. American Academy of Ophthalmology, pp. 77–139.

Rüschen, H., Celaschi, D., Bunce, C. and Carr, C. (2005). Randomised controlled trial of sub-Tenon's block versus topical anaesthesia for cataract surgery: a comparison of patient satisfaction. *Br. J. Ophthalmol.* **89**: 291–293.

6

Management of the patient with cataract and astigmatism

CK Patel

Introduction

It is useful at the outset to summarize the algorithmic approach to patient management developed in this chapter:

- Patients with astigmatism who develop cataract may also expect to enjoy the benefits of spectacle independence for distance vision in the same way as those without astigmatism.
- Avoid discussing correction of existing astigmatism with patients who have always worn spectacles and are perfectly at ease with the notion of continuing to wear spectacles post-operatively.
- Keratometry, performed as part of the biometry, will identify those patients with clinically significant astigmatism, e.g. >1.0 D cylinder (DC).
- For astigmatism between 1.0 and 4.0 DC there is the option of choosing either incisional techniques or a toric intraocular lens (IOL).
- For greater degrees of astigmatism, a standard spherical IOL at the time of cataract surgery followed by laser refractive surgery where suitable, as a second-stage procedure, is recommended.
- Biometry data should include anterior chamber depth and be plugged into nomograms for limbal relaxing incisions (LRI) or corneal relaxing incisions (CRI).

Optometrists are increasingly in the front line, making a diagnosis of cataract, initiating the process of informed consent and co-managing post-operative care with ophthalmologists. As such it is important to emphasize that modern cataract surgery is an operation not only to deal with the opaque lens but also to correct residual refractive error: the Holy Grail of spectacle-free vision for all distances, simulating the visual performance of the pre-presbyopic emmetropic eye, is increasingly being demanded by patients. The emphasis of this chapter is to discuss the practical issues relating to active management of combined cataract and regular astigmatism to achieve this goal. In-depth discussion of laser refractive techniques is beyond the scope of this chapter.

What is astigmatism?

Spherical refractive surfaces focus light equally in all directions onto the fovea in the emmetropic eye, and focus it in front or behind the fovea in myopia and hypermetropia, respectively. Astigmatism is an optical aberration in which refractive surfaces dissociate a point light source into different planes (Figure 6.1). Regular astigmatism is associated with two perpendicular planes and associated focal points. It is said to be with-the-rule (WTR) or against-the-rule (ATR) depending on whether the steep meridian is vertical or horizontal, respectively, with oblique astigmatism in-between. The optical nomenclature that describes the variation in positions of the principal foci relative to the fovea for WTR are given in Figure 6.2.

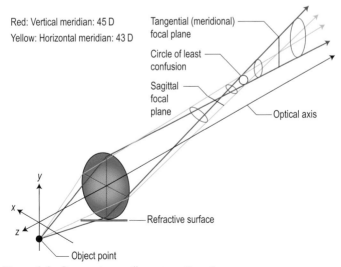

Figure 6.1 Ray tracing to illustrate astigmatism

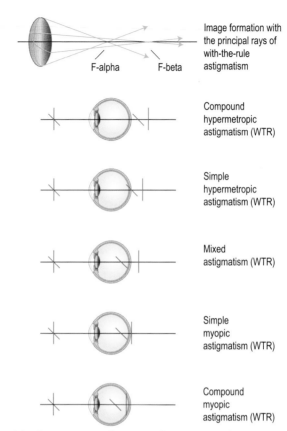

F-alpha   F-beta

Image formation with
the principal rays of
with-the-rule
astigmatism

Compound
hypermetropic
astigmatism (WTR)

Simple
hypermetropic
astigmatism (WTR)

Mixed
astigmatism (WTR)

Simple
myopic
astigmatism (WTR)

Compound
myopic
astigmatism (WTR)

Figure 6.2   Ray tracing to illustrate different types of WTR astigmatism

Astigmatism is a vector: it has magnitude and direction. Magnitude is measured in dioptres of cylinder (DC) and is the difference between maximal and minimal corneal power. Direction is better described as a meridian rather than an axis to avoid confusion when performing the surgical correction. In Figure 6.1, for example, the difference in corneal power between the red 90-degree meridian and flatter 180-degree meridian is:

$$45 \text{ D} - 43 \text{ D} = 2 \text{ D astigmatism.}$$

Assuming the spherical power of the refractive system is −3.00 dioptres sphere (DS), the spectacle prescription is written in minus and plus cylinder, as:

−3.00 DS/−2.00 DC × 180 (minus cylinder)
−5.00 DS/+2.00 DC × 90 (plus cylinder).

It can therefore be seen that a plus cylinder axis is equivalent to the steep meridian whereas the minus cylinder axis is equivalent to the flat meridian. It is vital that decimal points and signs are written clearly to minimize the risk of error.

The spectacle astigmatic prescription is composed of those due to anterior and posterior surfaces of both the cornea and the crystalline lens. That due to the posterior corneal surface and lens is minimal, but occasionally it can be clinically significant and so should be considered in the differential diagnosis of post-operative surprises in refractive outcome. Ocular surface incisions, tilt of intraocular lenses (IOLs) and rotation of toric implants all result in surgically induced astigmatism (SIA). With regard to incisions, the closer the incision is to the optical axis the greater the degree of SIA. Length and depth of incision also affect SIA.

In summary, the different types of astigmatism to consider are:

- **regular**: two focal points
- **irregular**: multiple focal points
- **with-the-rule**: steep meridian at 90 degrees
- **against-the-rule**: steep meridian at 180 degrees
- **oblique**: steep meridian at oblique angle
- **lenticular**: that part of refractive astigmatism attributed to crystalline lens
- **SIA**: secondary to surgical complications
  - tight sutures
  - tilt of IOLs
  - incorrect placement of LRI/CRI
  - incorrect placement of toric IOLs
  - post-operative rotation of toric IOLs.

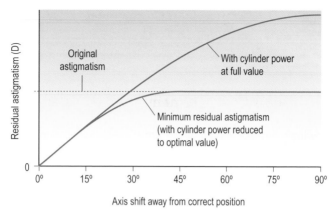

Figure 6.3 Axis misalignment versus residual astigmatism

Errors of axis alignment during surgical correction are an important contributor to SIA, but they are predictable according to the graph shown in Figure 6.3.

Misalignment of 10, 20 and 30 degrees reduces the correction by one-third, two-thirds and neutralizes the intended correction, respectively. Greater errors both induce cylinder and change the axis of astigmatism. A change in axis is clinically very disabling, especially if WTR or ATR astigmatism changes to an oblique position. This is because the fusion range compensating for image tilt, induced by oblique astigmatism, is limited.

How frequently is regular astigmatism encountered and what is its clinical impact?

Refractive astigmatism of 1.0, 2.0 and 3.0 DC reduce uncorrected Snellen visual acuity to 6/9 (20/30), 6/15 (20/50), 6/21–6/30 (20/70–20/100), respectively. Fifteen percent of patients undergoing cataract surgery have astigmatism greater than 1.0 D and represent the group for which it is generally worth considering astigmatic correction. Refraction and keratometry

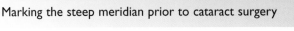
show that ATR astigmatism is the most common. However, corneal topography suggests that WTR astigmatism is under recognized. There is a tendency towards ATR change with age.

Pre-operative assessment

Following a decision to target the astigmatism during cataract surgery one needs an assessment of the magnitude and alignment of the astigmatism. Refractive astigmatism is a result of corneal and lenticular components. As cataract surgery will eliminate the lenticular component, the astigmatic target is based on assessment of the corneal component. The simplest method to measure the magnitude and direction of corneal astigmatism is to use keratometry. It is important to be consistent with nomenclature in order to avoid confusion: this chapter refers to meridians rather than axes when describing corneal power, noting that the two are perpendicular. Corneal topography if available is preferred to keratometry as it assesses corneal power over a wider area. Corneal topographers such as the Orbscan (Bausch and Lomb) also measure the power of posterior corneal surface, in addition to the anterior surface, and hence can detect those rare cases where the posterior corneal surface significantly contributes to the astigmatic error. Many topography systems also estimate corneal thickness and are helpful in planning incisional refractive surgery. The disadvantage is the extra cost involved.

Marking the steep meridian prior to cataract surgery

For combined phacoemulsification and astigmatic correction, reference points on the cornea or limbus to identify the steep corneal meridian need to be recognized while the patient is lying down on the operating table. Head tilt is associated with ocular torsion and it is therefore regarded as essential to mark the reference points with a patient vertical and fixing a target that is level with the eyes; this can either be at a slit lamp or seated on an operating trolley. One option is to use reference points on the iris such as focal naevi or crypts. In practice the author rarely finds this method useful as pupil dilation and complications such as iris prolapse have the potential to result in error in identifying such reference points.

The author's preferred method (Figure 6.4) is to seat the patient in the anaesthetic room, fixing a target that is level with the eyes. Topical anaesthetic drops are applied. A spear is used to expose and dry the inferior limbus and a marker pen is used to estimate the 6 o'clock reference position. One has to be quick in exposing a dry area and marking it between blinks as the ink tends to spread on a wet surface. Next, the upper lid is similarly retracted and a 12 o'clock reference position marked. It may be useful for an assistant to retract the lower lid so that the 6 o'clock mark is visible. The horizontal reference points are then marked. Under the operating microscope additional marks can be applied in the relevant quadrants to denote 30-degree (1 clock hour) increments. The marks should be as close to the cornea as possible as perilimbal conjunctiva is least likely to translocate if chemosis occurs when sub-Tenons anaesthetic is applied. For this reason most surgeons prefer topical anaesthesia for cataract surgery. It should then be possible to estimate with a fair degree of accuracy the location of the steep meridian, which should be marked on a pre-operative proforma. A more expensive option is to purchase surgical protractors.

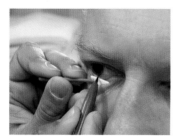 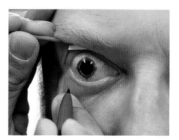

Figure 6.4 Marking the steep meridian prior to cataract surgery

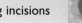
On-axis incisions

For patients where corneal astigmatism is less than 1.0 DC it is important to minimize SIA. Contemporary corneal and limbal incisions less than 2.75 mm in width are said to be 'astigmatically neutral'. However, it is prudent, but not essential, to place the incision on the steepest meridian. This would be an advantage if there were accidental extension of the incision or if wound burn occurs, which has the potential of contributing adversely to SIA. There are two approaches to achieving consistent placement of incisions on-axis: either a surgeon has to learn to perform cataract surgery and be prepared to use the phacoemulsification probe with the non-dominant hand so as to always be able to place the incision on-axis and still remain at the head of the table, or the surgeon has to perform phacoemulsification always using the dominant hand (the preferences of the vast majority of cataract surgeons) and operate seated either at the side or head of the table.

Limbal relaxing and corneal relaxing incisions

Wound behaviour following a partial thickness unsutured incision, made parallel to the limbus, flattens the meridian perpendicular to the direction of the incision. This reduces the power of the cornea in that meridian, but through a process known as coupling it increases the power in the perpendicular meridian. For limbal relaxing incisions (LRIs) this coupling can safely be assumed to be 1:1, and the implication is that the spherical target for the biometry is independent of the astigmatic changes induced by surgery. For corneal relaxing incisions (CRIs) this may not be the case.

Method

Either the steepest or flattest meridians need to be marked, as previously described. Several decisions need to be made and documented clearly so that the risk of error at the time of surgery is reduced.

Incisions for phacoemulsification instrumentation

Phaco-probe and side-port incisions are considered astigmatically neutral, and it is necessary to decide the merits of separating or incorporating the LRI from or into the probe wound. The author's preference is to separate the probe wound from keratotomy as theoretically the surgeon may extend the probe wound more than planned during insertion of an implant. The author has not experienced any difficulty with incorporating side-port incisions into an LRI.

CRIs versus LRIs

CRIs are performed at optical zones of 8–9 mm and are therefore closer to the visual axis in comparison with LRIs. The astigmatic correction for equivalent wound healing effect is therefore greater for CRIs than LRIs. The general view, however, is that there is less variability with LRIs and a lower risk of overcorrection and axis misalignment in comparison with CRIs. CRIs are associated with a risk of glare, especially with an enlarged scotopic pupil. A 1:1 coupling is also more likely with LRIs and means that the spherical IOL power does not need to be adjusted.

Incision characteristics

Wound healing determines the effect of any incision and it is therefore not a surprise that incision characteristics are determined by age and location of incision with respect to visual axis (LRIs versus CRIs). The astigmatic range that can be corrected by incisional refractive surgery varies from 0.5 D to 8.0 D, with LRIs able to deliver 0.5–4.0 DC of correction. These variables are used in nomograms to inform the answer to the first three questions posed.

Variable or fixed-depth guarded knives are required for incisions. Guarded diamond knives are popular but expensive. Fixed-depth knives may be cheaper and more convenient to use. An instrument to fix the cornea while the incision is made, such as the modified Fine-Thornton ring, is essential. The depth of the incision must be even and is critical to the astigmatic correction; it should be performed on a firm globe. The LRIs should therefore be performed first. For most patients, a blade setting of 600 μm is used; however, a blade setting of 500–575 μm is recommended for patients older than 80 years and for those patients with corneoscleral thinning. LRIs are placed in the steep axis at the limbus, just anterior to the palisades of Vogt. A 6-mm incision is required for each diopter of astigmatism up to 2 DC; to correct astigmatism between 2 and 3 DC, LRIs of 8 mm in length may be used. For astigmatism greater than 4 DC, LRIs are combined with CRIs to attain adequate correction. Compared with older patients, younger patients require longer incisions to achieve the same effect. When used, CRIs are at 99% depth at the 8- or 9-mm optical zone, 2 mm in length for every dioptre over 4 D.

The author then performs the main phacoemulsification incision, followed by inflation of anterior chamber with a viscoelastic, and then side-port incisions. The remainder of the phacoemulsification procedure does not need to be modified.

Relative contraindications

Relative contraindications for LRI include:

- severe dry eye
- active corneal disease
- uncontrolled glaucoma.

Advantages of LRIs

Advantages

LRIs are easy to perform with a modest increase in reference costs.

Disadvantages

There is variability of effect. Extra incisions have the potential for structurally weakening the cornea, with attendant predisposition to globe rupture with trauma. There may also be a greater risk of early or delayed corneal infection, which can present with the following features:

- painful photophobic eye, with or without reduced corrected vision
- corneal infiltrate and oedema over LRI/CRI
- anterior chamber cells that can form a hypopyon.

If a corneal abscess is suspected then the patient should be advised to see an ophthalmologist as an emergency to receive aggressive antibiotic treatment following a diagnostic corneal scrape. The differential diagnosis of early corneal abscess is wound burn if the phaco incision and LRIs/CRIs are coaxial. A suture should not be removed prematurely in a patient with wound burn.

Microperforation is another complication that requires suturing, with suture removal 4 weeks later.

Post-operative asssessment

Specific differences in managing patients who undergo LRI/CRI are to monitor for signs of corneal abscess and to perform Siedel tests over the incisions in cases where there is hypotony or a shallow anterior chamber. If positive then use of a bandage contact lens could be considered.

Toric intraocular lens

An astigmatic correction can be built into the spherical component of an IOL, as it is with a spectacle lens. This concept is not new. Toric poly(methyl methacrylate) (PMMA) IOLs were developed in the past for use in patients presenting with cataract and post-corneal-graft astigmatism. These were large diameter rigid lenses and were therefore not ideal as large wounds were required for their insertion. SIA would therefore have affected the post-operative result. Several toric IOLs are now marketed in both foldable and injectable platforms.

The ideal toric intraocular lens

The general requirements of a toric lens are the same as those of any IOL:

- easy to fold
- easy to insert
- injectable option
- low rate of posterior capsule opacification.

The additional requirements specific to a toric lens are:

- easy to rotate during surgery
- easy to identify toric axis
- good IOL centration (decentration and tilt can induce astigmatism)
- good rotational stability during early and late post-operative periods
- stability maintained following YAG laser capsulotomy
- stability maintained following vitrectomy for retinal detachment.

Staar Surgical was the first to market a plate haptic toric lens made of silicone. Human Optics introduced a three-piece silicone toric IOL with serrated PMMA haptics. Rayner has recently marketed an acrylic toric lens based on the Center*flex* design (Figure 6.5), and Alcon is set to launch a toric lens based on the single-piece AcrySof platform. The Artiflex lens is an iris fixated foldable toric implant designed for phacic

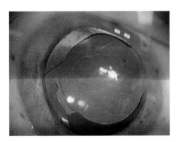

Figure 6.5 Rayner Center*flex* toric IOL

patients that has the potential to be used in patients where capsular bag or sulcus fixation of conventional toric IOLs is not possible.

In the author's experience, the trailing haptic of the Human Optics toric IOL requires a technique for insertion that differs from conventional loop haptics and may cause some difficulty when the implant is first used.

The plate haptic silicone platform is not ideal with respect to post-operative rotational stability, especially in the early post-operative period. The IOL has been modified, first by making it longer (from 10.80 mm to 11.20 mm) for a 'tighter' fit and second by introducing holes in the haptics, the theory being that capsular fusion locks the lens in place. Early post-operative rotation still appears to be a problem in some cases, requiring post-operative repositioning. The loop haptic three-piece platform made from silicone theoretically has a greater risk of late post-operative rotation.

The Rayner toric and AcrySof platforms have good early rotational stability track records.

Biometry for toric lenses

The objective is to calculate the spherical and cylindrical power of the implant. Note that the IOL cylindrical power will be greater than the spectacle cylinder because the IOL is closer to the nodal point of the eye.

Many IOL manufacturers prefer surgeons to use their calculation services, which involves exchanging biometry proformas by fax or electronically.

The spherical power of the lens can be calculated by assuming that the average K value is equivalent to the K value of the steepest meridian and by using the standard IOL power calculation equations. The spherical power is also calculated assuming an average K value equivalent to the flattest meridian. The difference between spherical power obtained from the steepest and flattest K values represents the astigmatic power of the implant required.

Method

Local banks of toric IOLs are not cost effective. One should make sure that systems are in place that ensure that two lenses from the manufacturer's bank are available in theatre, with the appropriate injectors and folders, before the patient arrives for surgery. The cornea is marked pre-operatively as discussed above. Care should be taken not to make the phacoemulsification wound too 'corneal' as SIA may affect the optical result. The capsulorrhexis should be circular and 1 mm less than the size of the IOL optic. Once the IOL is inserted, the author's preference is to place a single 10/0 nylon or vicryl wound suture for all cases, remove all viscoelastic, and then use the bimanual irrigation and aspiration to align the IOL to the appropriate meridian. The side ports can then be hydrated before removing the speculum. The suture is placed to avoid flux of fluid from the anterior chamber during removal of the speculum, which could result in movement of the IOL, especially in patients with large capsular bags.

In cases where the astigmatic correction is greater than 5 D one should try and use a surgical keratometer to confirm optimal IOL alignment. Piggyback toric IOLs have been used in the past to correct high degrees of astigmatism when customized cylinder corrections were not available. The IOLs needed to be sutured together to avoid independent movement.

Most toric IOLs are designed for capsular fixation. If a posterior capsule is breeched during surgery the first aim should be to try and convert it into a posterior continuous curvilinear capsulorrhexis (PCCC). This can then be followed by anterior vitrectomy and bag fixation of loop haptic toric IOLs. The silicone plate haptic toric IOL should not be used as there is a high risk of late dislocation into the vitreous. If a PCCC is not possible then anterior vitrectomy and clearance of soft lens matter should be completed. The patient could than have a conventional spherical IOL fixated in the posterior sulcus, with subsequent spectacle correction of cylinder or CRI/LRI. The alternative is to leave the patient aphakic and to consider the use of a secondary iris-fixated toric IOL.

Advantages and disadvantages of toric IOLs

Advantages
Toric IOLs have the advantage that the results are more predictable than for keratotomy. There is no added risk of corneal infection. The procedure is reversible, and if there is axis misalignment post-operatively it can be rectified.

Disadvantages
The option is more expensive, especially if the IOL is not a stock item and has to be custom built. Post-operative IOL rotation may compromise the result and require reoperation.

Post-operative assessment

Specific management goals are to dilate the pupil to check for IOL alignment when the refraction indicates a significant undercorrection or overcorrection with a change in axis. If the IOL has moved, it is easier to realign the IOL within 1 month of surgery, before the capsule is too firmly fused with the implant.

Combining toric IOLs and incisional techniques

This strategy has been used with success to reduce the number of incisions required when the cylindrical corrections with toric IOLs were limited.

Laser

Laser is an alternative to incisional techniques and toric IOLs, however it is largely available only in the private sector in the UK. It shares the same risks of corneal infection as keratotomy and is not reversible.

Future developments

Post-operative adjustment of the contour of IOLs can be used to adjust the spherical component of a patient's refraction. If this

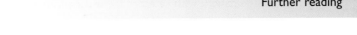
light-adjustable technology can be modified for orientation-specific adjustment, the result would be the ultimate toric IOL. However, this will clearly come at a high price.

Further reading

Gills, J.P. (2002). Treating astigmatism at the time of cataract surgery. *Curr. Opin. Ophthalmol.* **13**:2–6.

Lindstrom, R.L, Koch, D.D., Osher, R.H. and Wang, L. (2004). Control of astigmatism in the cataract patient.
In: *Cataract Surgery: technique, complications, and management*, 2nd edition: Ed: Steinert, R.F. Saunders, Chapter 22.

Woodcock, M., Shah, S. and Smith, R.J. (2004). Recent advances in customising cataract surgery. *BMJ* **328**(3): 92–96.

7

Post-operative management following cataract surgery

Manoj V Parulekar

Introduction

Cataract surgery is increasingly performed as a daycase procedure with infrequent review. Much of the care pathway may be undertaken by properly trained and supervised non-medical members of the team, including nurses, technicians and optometrists. Knowledge of the normal post-operative timescale for recovery allows a clinician to detect abnormalities early in order to instigate timely and appropriate intervention.

As volume of surgery increases and personnel other than ophthalmologists are involved in post-operative follow-up, it is increasingly recognized that guidelines for the efficient management of routine as well as more complicated cases are required in order to help minimize inappropriate delay in any required post-operative intervention.

As a general rule, a full dilated slit-lamp examination at 1 month, following even routine uneventful cataract surgery and final cessation of medication for example, helps identify potential sight-threatening complications and should be considered the benchmark for post-operative follow-up.

While there may be variations in practice, the basic principles of routine post-operative management of cataract patients remain unchanged. This chapter deals with the principles of management after routine uncomplicated cataract surgery and considers certain special situations.

Following uncomplicated cataract surgery

Eye pad/shield

Most surgeons would cover the operated eye with a pad and shield for a few hours following surgery under peribulbar or sub-Tenon's anaesthesia due to the possibility of persistent corneal anaesthesia and the lack of a blink reflex or Bell's phenomenon.

A shield alone may be sufficient after surgery using topical anaesthesia. It is prudent to place a pad and shield over the eye at

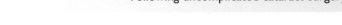
the end of general anaesthesia in order to avoid accidental injury during awaking.

It is advisable to protect the eye with a shield at night for approximately 2 weeks after surgery to prevent accidental injury during sleep.

Acetazolamide

Oral acetazolamide may be used post-operatively by some surgeons to prevent post-operative intraocular pressure spikes within the first 12 hours after surgery. While individual preference varies, the sustained release preparation is commonly used: 250 mg, 12 hourly for up to 1 day after surgery.

Patients may experience tingling (pins and needles sensation), tiredness and loss of appetite after taking acetazolamide and should be warned of these potential side effects, which may occur within 24 hours following surgery.

Analgesia

It is unusual to experience significant pain or discomfort after routine uncomplicated cataract surgery.

Minor discomfort and pain can be controlled with oral paracetamol: 500–1000 mg, 6 hourly. Ibuprofen can be used for moderate pain: 400 mg, 8 hourly.

Extreme pain should alert the observer to the possibility of a corneal abrasion, wound leak with iris prolapse or suprachoroidal haemorrhage. Slit-lamp and fundus examinations should be performed if unexpected pain is experienced.

Post-operative check

The first-day post-operative review is no longer in widespread use, and many ophthalmic departments have replaced this with a routine telephone call by a trained nurse. It is, however, routine practice in some units to review patients 1–2 hours post-operatively before discharge, and on the first post-operative day in other units.

A first-day post-operative visit may be required:

- where surgery was complicated
- with coexisting eye disease, e.g. glaucoma, uveitis
- for patients with an only eye.

Robust arrangements need to be in place to ensure that patients not reviewed the next day after routine cataract surgery have easy access to advice and assessment, and that post-operative complications can be identified and managed quickly. If the post-operative management is shared with nurses, optometrists or orthoptists working within the unit, or by accredited optometrists working outside the unit, it is important for them to have access to an ophthalmologist for advice.

Telephone assessment
The benchmark information to obtain and protocol during the first-day post-operative telephone assessment following routine cataract surgery should be as follows:

1. How much can the patient can see? Any improvement or reduction in vision?
   - distance—e.g. see clock
   - near—e.g. pick up newspaper
2. Are there any visual disturbances?
3. Advise patient to note how red the eye is now and that if any increase in redness occurs they should contact eye department.
4. Is there any pain, discomfort or sensitivity to light?
5. Is there any eyelid swelling?
6. Is there any discharge?
7. Are there any problems using eye drops?
8. Remind the patient on how to use eye drops.
9. Inform the ophthalmologist if any complications or concerns are highlighted.

Post-operative examination
At the same-day or following-day post-operative examination, it is necessary to look at the following:

1. The **wound**: the integrity of the wound should be checked with the Seidel test, where a drop of 2% fluorescein is instilled into the conjunctival sac and the wound examined under a blue light (cobalt blue filter of the slit lamp). Any leak of aqueous would show up as a clear dark stream diluting the green stained tear film. Other things to look for include phacoemulsification corneal wound burns and the presence of a suture (Figure 7.1). If there is a suture, look for exposed or protruding suture ends that may require rotating so that the knot is buried into the corneal stroma.

2. The **anterior chamber**: the depth of the anterior chamber must be assessed. An excessively shallow anterior chamber should prompt a careful search for a wound leak (see above). If the anterior chamber is excessively deep, it may be advisable

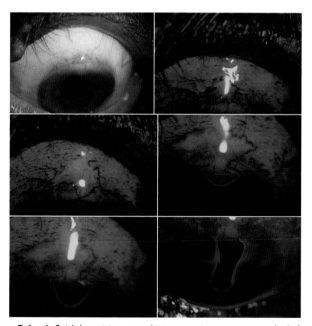

Figure 7.1 A Seidel-positive test, demonstrating an aqueous leak from a corneal wound that was complicated by a burn and required sutures. The clear dark stream of aqueous fluid dilutes the green stained tear film

to check for a dislocated intraocular lens (IOL) position or high intraocular pressure (IOP). The degree of cellular activity in the anterior chamber should be estimated, and the presence of fibrin or blood should be recorded.

3. The **clarity of the cornea**: an excessively cloudy cornea should be reported.
4. The **position of the IOL**: any malposition of the IOL should be reported immediately.
5. The **shape of the pupil**: a misshapen pupil may indicate iris capture within the wound, surgical trauma or distortion of the pupil by vitreous or a displaced IOL.

It is particularly important to measure the IOP after complicated surgery or combined cataract and glaucoma or vitreo-retinal surgery. Post-operative IOP spikes can occur due to retained viscoelastic material in the anterior chamber and require medication.

The measurement of visual acuity soon after surgery is of limited value as it may be affected by corneal clarity, inflammation and the effect of local anaesthesia on optic nerve function.

Instructions at discharge

An important component of post-operative management is instructing the patients prior to discharge. The patients should be told what to expect over the ensuing weeks, with full explanation of warning signs and how to seek help and arrange an urgent review if they are concerned.

Indications of complications

Findings at discharge on the day of routine cataract surgery that should alert to the possibility of a complication include:

- a leaky wound or shallow anterior chamber
- excessive corneal oedema (a cloudy cornea)
- blood, fibrin or lens matter in the anterior chamber
- a malpositioned IOL
- an abnormally shaped pupil.

What should a patient expect

The patient should be given a clear explanation of the surgery they have undergone, and it should be stressed that while it may seem a relatively routine procedure, careful observation of instructions is important to a successful outcome. Some degree of anxiety is expected, which can be minimized by giving written instructions in clear language in large print. These simple measures can significantly reduce patient's anxiety.

- **Pain**: it is unusual to experience pain after cataract surgery, although some discomfort may be expected for a few days after. Severe pain should warrant referral for examination.
- **Improvement in vision**: the improvement in vision is incremental over the first few days or weeks after surgery and should be sustained. Any deterioration in vision should be reported immediately. If the desired refractive result is emmetropia, the unaided distance vision in the operated eye is expected to be reasonable, although spectacle correction will be needed by a significant number of patients to achieve sharp vision for both far distance and reading. This would have been explained pre-operatively, and could be reiterated post-operatively to avoid unnecessary visits by anxious patients.
- **Redness**: some redness and light sensitivity may persist for a few days, but it should progressively improve.
- **Watering**: some watering may occur for a few days. Excessive watering may indicate a leaky wound and should be reported.

RSVP

The combination of:

- **R**edness
- **S**ensitivity to light
- **V**isual disturbance or deterioration, and
- **P**ain

is ominous and warrants urgent assessment, particularly to exclude endophthalmitis.

Daily activities following cataract surgery

- **Diet**: no dietary restrictions are needed after cataract surgery.
- **Resuming work and physical activities**: it is advisable to avoid heavy activity for up to 4 weeks after cataract surgery. It is, however, reasonable to continue routine activities at home, such as cooking, and to resume desk jobs within a few days of surgery. There are no restrictions on bending after routine phacoemulsification cataract surgery.
- **Bathing, showering and swimming**: wound healing occurs rapidly after surgery, achieving stability between 7 and 60 days after surgery (mean 4 weeks). Showering and bathing may be resumed a few days after surgery, taking care to avoid water entering the eye. Swimming should be avoided for 4 weeks after surgery.
- **Driving**: it is reasonable to resume driving within days of cataract surgery if the operated or fellow eye fulfils the legal visual requirements for driving (visual acuity and fields). It is advisable to allow for a period of adjustment after surgery to get accustomed to the new situation, particularly in cases of anisometropia. The Driver and Vehicle Licensing Agency (DVLA) guidelines are:

> Any decision regarding returning to driving must take into account several issues. These include recovery from the surgical procedure, recovery from anaesthesia, the distracting effect of pain, impairment due to analgesia (sedation and cognitive impairment) as well as any physical restrictions due to the surgery, underlying condition or other co-morbid conditions. It is the responsibility of the driver to ensure that he/she is in control of the vehicle at all times and to be able to demonstrate that is so, if stopped by the police. It might also be reasonable for the driver to check his/her insurance policy before returning to drive after surgery.

Medications

Topical anti-inflammatory agents are routinely used after cataract surgery to control post-operative inflammation. Most surgeons use topical steroids (dexamethasone 0.1% or prednisolone actetate 0.5 or 1%), while some use non-steroidal agents (ketorolac 0.5%). The usual frequency is four times a day, for

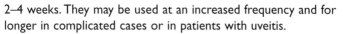
2–4 weeks. They may be used at an increased frequency and for longer in complicated cases or in patients with uveitis.

In cases where the patient or carer may experience difficulty instilling drops at the required frequency, ointment may be used at a reduced frequency (twice a day).

The role of topical antibiotics post-operatively in the prevention of endophthalmitis is unproven. However, a significant proportion of surgeons will prescribe topical antibiotics for 1–4 weeks after surgery. This may be as a combined antibiotic steroid preparation for convenience.

The patient should be advised to wash hands prior to instilling drops, and to avoid touching the eye or lashes with the tip of the bottle.

Cleaning the eye

The patient should be instructed to clean the eyelids with boiled water and sterile cotton wool, taking care to avoid water entering the eye.

Final review

A review appointment is necessary to:

- review progress and medication
- assess the visual and refractive outcome and collect data
- identify any problems or complications
- discuss second-eye surgery where appropriate
- arrange follow-up for coexisting eye disease
- provide advice on spectacle prescription (which can be prescribed approximately 4 weeks following phacoemulsification).

This examination can be provided by an ophthalmologist, nurse, optometrist or orthoptist working within the unit, or by an accredited optometrist working outside the unit (both in accordance with agreed guidelines). The ophthalmologist with responsibility for the patient should ensure that appropriate training and monitoring takes place when the post-operative care is delegated to others.

Timing of the final review

Several studies have demonstrated that the refraction stabilizes between 1 and 2 weeks after surgery. However, the timing of the final post-operative visit should be at approximately 4–6 weeks after surgery. This would allow assessment of both the refractive outcome and any complications, such as cystoid macular oedema (CMO), persistent or recurrent post-operative uveitis and early posterior capsular opacification.

What should be carried out at the final review

It is mandatory to perform a thorough eye examination at this visit:

- Unaided and pinhole visual acuity must be checked, and also the autorefraction.
- IOP should be recorded.
- The state of the cornea and wound must be noted. Sutures from phacoemulsification wounds can ordinarily be removed at this visit by an ophthalmologist, however there are certain situations where sutures should be left for longer, including:
  - conversion to extracapsular cataract extraction
  - corneal wound burn.

In such cases, the decision to remove sutures should be left to the ophthalmologist.

- Centration of the IOL implant and opacification of the posterior capsule should be recorded.
- The anterior chamber should show little or no activity at this visit. Uveitis with 1+ cells or 2+ cells seen within a 2×2 mm field should be notified to the ophthalmologist.
- A dilated slit-lamp fundus examination should be carried out as routine, particularly for patients with high myopia, diabetic retinopathy or macular degeneration.

If the final review is being carried out by an optometrist, the following should alert the need for referral back to the ophthalmologist:

- The patient gives a history of pain, discomfort or sudden reduction in vision.

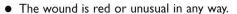

- The wound is red or unusual in any way.
- Intolerable or unacceptable astigmatism.
- Intolerable or unacceptable anisometropia.
- Corrected acuity is worse than pre-operatively, has decreased post-operatively or is less than 6/12.
- Raised IOP, either in comparison with the other eye or with pre-operative measurements.
- Examination unable to be carried out.
- Slit lamp examination findings of:
  - anterior chamber activity present (more than two cells seen in 2×2 mm field)
  - cornea not clear
  - posterior synechiae
  - thickening of the posterior capsule
  - any vitreous activity
  - any loose or protruding suture.

Refractive changes and stability

The final visit is very useful for assessing the refractive and visual outcome of surgery. Any persistent astigmatism or ametropia will be evident at this visit. Excessive ametropia should be reported as well as excessive induced astigmatism.

As a general rule, induced astigmatism greater than 2 D and unexpected ametropia greater than 1–2 D should be considered significant as it is likely to affect the unaided visual acuity.

Anisometropia and second-eye surgery

In cases with high hypermetropia or myopia, emmetropia is often the desired refractive outcome. This would inevitably result in bothersome anisometropia following first-eye surgery and necessitate expedited surgery for the other eye.

Complications at the final review

Complaints of photophobia, a tender and red eye or blurry vision at the final visit can be due to cystoid macular oedema or low grade endophthalmitis, and should prompt referral to the ophthalmologist.

> **Second-eye surgery**
>
> The final review provides the opportunity to examine and discuss the need and timing of surgery for the second eye.

Complicated and difficult situations

Combined cataract and glaucoma or vitreo-retinal surgery

All such cases should be seen by the ophthalmologist.

Diabetes

There is an increased risk of progression of retinopathy, especially maculopathy, after cataract surgery. Any patient with known maculopathy or moderate non-proliferative diabetic retinopathy should therefore be seen by an ophthalmologist for examination within 3 months of cataract surgery.

Evidence suggests that the risk of new-onset macular oedema in diabetics may be reduced by the use of non-steroidal anti-inflammatory agents such as topical ketorolac (Voltarol or Acular) four times a day for 4 weeks following surgery.

Uveitis

Any history of previous uveitis increases the risk of persistent uveitis and CMO following routine cataract surgery. Topical steroids may have to be increased in both frequency and duration.

Some surgeons administer a sub-Tenon's steroid injection either prior to or immediately following surgery in patients with a history of recurrent uveitis. In such cases it is important to monitor the IOP as steroid-induced pressure rise can occur several months after the injection.

All patients with a history of uveitis who are undergoing cataract surgery should be seen for review by the ophthalmologist.

Glaucoma

Patients with advanced glaucoma are at increased risk of optic nerve damage from post-operative spikes in IOP. The prophylactic use of acetazolamide (or topical IOP-lowering agents) for 2–3 days post-operatively is highly recommended in such cases.

Patients with pre-existing glaucoma are also at increased risk of a steroid-induced rise in IOP. The risk however is small for short courses of topical steroids. Careful attention should be paid to IOP measurement at the final review, and the patient referred to the ophthalmologist if the IOP is elevated.

Patients who are on antiglaucoma medications should be advised to continue taking them following cataract surgery. This is true for all medications except the prostaglandin analogues (e.g. latanoprost, bimatoprost and travaprost), the use of which may increase the risk of developing post-operative CMO. The use of these medications should be discussed with the ophthalmologist, who can assess the risk of CMO and advise a temporary change or cessation of medication if required.

Age-related macular degeneration

It is well recognized that patients with age-related macular degeneration (ARMD) undergoing cataract surgery are at increased risk of progression of maculopathy, including conversion

---

Glaucoma patients

- Patients on antiglaucoma medications should continue them post-operatively.
- Patients undergoing combined cataract and glaucoma surgery will be advised by the ophthalmologist to discontinue antiglaucoma medications in most cases.
- Prostaglandin analogues **may** be discontinued by individual surgeons in certain circumstances for a few weeks following surgery.

of dry (non-exudative) to wet (exudative) ARMD. This increase in risk persists for months to years after surgery. While all patients need not be seen by an ophthalmologist at final review, they should be asked to report back promptly if they notice any deterioration in central vision. There is some evidence that periocular (intravitreal) steroid injection may reduce the risk of progression, and it is used routinely by some surgeons. In such cases, the IOP should be monitored for up to 6 months after surgery due to the risk of steroid-induced glaucoma.

Other corneal pathology

Any patients with coexistent corneal disease should ideally be seen by an ophthalmologist. This particularly applies to endothelial dystrophy. Stable corneal opacities may not require a review by an ophthalmologist.

Patients with pre-existing herpetic eye disease may experience a flare-up of the epithelial disease following surgery. This could be due to local trauma, surgical stress or the use of steroids post-operatively. Such cases may receive prophylactic topical acyclovir eye ointment from the ophthalmologist. Any suspicion of reactivation of herpetic eye disease should prompt urgent referral to the ophthalmologist.

Herpetic eye disease

Any suspicion of reactivation of herpetic eye disease should prompt urgent referral to the ophthalmologist.

Other retinal pathology

Patients may report new-onset floaters or flashing lights following cataract surgery. This may be due to posterior vitreous detachment. Such cases should be referred to the ophthalmologist for a dilated retinal examination to exclude retinal tears.

Complications during surgery

All such cases (e.g. posterior capsular rupture) should be seen by the ophthalmologist. These patients may receive topical steroid treatment at an increased frequency, and for longer than routine cases (see Chapter 8).

Further reading

Ahmed, I.I., Kranemann, C., Chipman, M. and Malam, F. (2002). Revisiting early postoperative follow-up after phacoemulsification. *J. Cataract. Refract. Surg.* **28**(1): 100–108.

Barba, K.R., Samy, A., Lai, C., Perlman, J.I. and Bouchard, C.S. (2000). Effect of topical anti-inflammatory drugs on corneal and limbal wound healing. *J. Cataract. Refract. Surg.* **26**(6): 893–897.

DVLA Drivers Medical Group (2007). *At a Glance Guide to the Current Medical Standards of Fitness to Drive.* DVLA, Chapter 6. www.dvla.gov.uk/medical/ataglance.aspx.

Hirneiss, C., Neubauer, A.S., Kampik, A. and Schonfeld, C.L. (2005). Comparison of prednisolone 1%, rimexolone 1% and ketorolac tromethamine 0.5% after cataract extraction: a prospective, randomized, double-masked study. *Graefe's Arch. Clin. Exp. Ophthalmol.* **243**(8): 768–773.

Lake, D., Fong, K. and Wilson, R. (2005). Early refractive stabilization after temporal phacoemulsification: what is the optimum time for spectacle prescription? *J. Cataract Refract. Surg.* **31**(9):1845.

The Royal College of Ophthalmologists (2004). *Cataract Surgery Guidelines.* www.rcophth.ac.uk/about/publications.

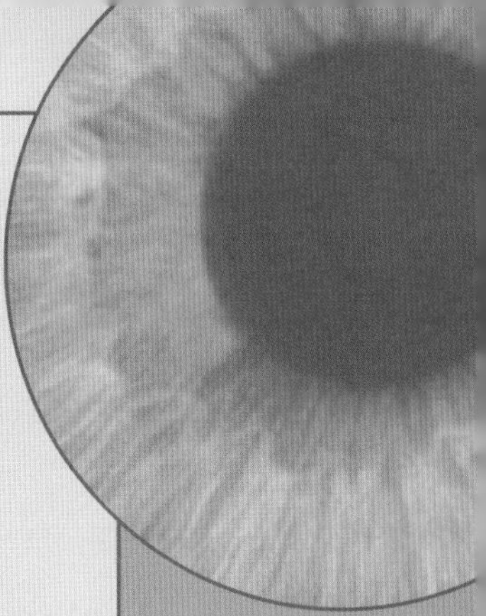

8 Complications following cataract surgery

Manoj V Parulekar

contents continue

8
Complications following cataract surgery

Manoj V Parulekar

Cataract surgery remains the most frequently performed elective procedure across the world. It has evolved over the years into a very safe and effective procedure, affording quick rehabilitation. It is, however, important to remember that despite being variously described as 'routine', 'straightforward', 'simple' or even 'minor', cataract surgery still remains a highly demanding technical exercise. Complications may be few and relatively infrequent, but the margin for error is very small, and this seemingly straightforward operation may potentially result in complete loss of vision.

Complications occurring and manifesting during surgery have been dealt with in Chapter 5. This chapter focuses on the various complications that could manifest or occur post-operatively. These complications are summarized in the boxes below in terms of timing of onset and frequency of incidence.

Wound-related complications

Wound leak

Incidence
Infrequent.

Symptoms
Excessive watering from the eye, with or without blurred vision.

Causes
Too short a corneal tunnel, a poorly constructed wound, excessively large wounds and phaco wound burns (thermal injury to the corneal lip during phacoemulsification, typically seen with dense cataracts).

Examination findings
The Seidel test would be positive in most cases; aqueous will leak from the wound leak site diluting the fluorescein in the tear film. (Figure 7.1 shows a Seidel-positive test, demonstrating an occult aqueous leak from a corneal wound that was complicated by a burn and required sutures. Application of 2% fluorescein causes a

Incidence of complications

- **Common (up to 10% of cases):**
  - raised intraocular pressure (IOP)
  - corneal oedema
  - posterior capsular opacification (PCO)
  - induced astigmatism
  - ametropia
  - posterior vitreous detachment (PVD)
  - acetozolamide adverse effects
- **Infrequent (up to 5% of cases):**
  - wound leak
  - persistent uveitis
  - suture irritation
  - cystoid macular oedema (CMO)
  - progression of coexistent retinal disease
  - conjunctival chemosis
  - allergy to topical medications
- **Rare (approximately 1% of cases):**
  - recurrent uveitis
  - corneal wound burn
  - corneal abrasion
  - retained lens matter
  - steroid-induced glaucoma
  - glare effect
- **Very rare (less than 1% of cases):**
  - iris defects
  - ptosis
  - diplopia
  - endophthalmitis
  - vitreous wick
  - iris prolapse
  - endothelial damage
  - Descemet detachment
  - closed suprachoroidal haemorrhage
  - hyphaema
  - IOL decentration
  - IOL haptic prolapse
  - phimosis of anterior capsule
  - retinal tear or detachment

Onset of complications

The approximate time following cataract surgery when typical post-operative complications are identified:

- **Early (1–3 days):**
  - wound leak
  - conjunctival chemosis
  - corneal abrasion
  - corneal wound burn
  - hyphaema
  - corneal oedema
  - raised intraocular pressure (IOP)
  - intraocular lens (IOL) haptic prolapse
  - iris prolapse
  - suprachoroidal haemorrhage
  - Descemet detachment
  - acetazolamide adverse effects
  - endophthalmitis
- **Intermediate (1–2 weeks)**
  - corneal oedema
  - Descemet detachment
  - suture irritation
  - preservative or drug allergy
  - retained lens matter
  - endophthalmitis
  - ametropia
  - posterior vitreous detachment (PVD)
- **Late (3–4 weeks):**
  - posterior capsular opacification (PCO)
  - cystoid macular oedema (CMO)
  - endophthalmitis
  - persistent uveitis
  - induced astigmatism
- **Delayed (after 1 month):**
  - IOL decentration
  - glare effect
  - PCO
  - low-grade endophthalmitis
  - recurrent uveitis
  - diplopia

Continued

- **Delayed (after 1 month):—cont'd**
  - corneal endothelial damage
  - glare effect
  - anisometropia
  - ptosis
  - retinal tear or detachment
  - PVD
  - progression of coexistent retinal disease
  - steroid-induced glaucoma (if steroids are continued).

stream of aqueous to fluoresce bright green when viewed under cobalt blue light, indicating a positive Seidel test result.)

However, there are situations where the Seidel test may be negative despite the presence of a leak. This could happen if a considerable amount of aqueous has already been lost and the anterior chamber is very shallow, or with an intermittent leak. Wound leaks can occur despite the presence of a corneal suture.

Importance
There is an increased risk of endophthalmitis, contact between the intraocular lens (IOL) and the corneal endothelium, uveitis and iris prolapse in the presence of a wound leak.

Management
Seek urgent ophthalmic advice. Small leaks may be observed with topical antibiotic prophylaxis, particularly if the anterior chamber is formed. Pad overnight or bandage contact lens for persistent or brisk leaks. Corneal wound suturing if the anterior chamber is shallow, especially if the leak is brisk. This should be done urgently if there is risk of endothelial touch or in the presence of iris prolapse, but it can be deferred to the following day if the anterior chamber is shallow but formed.

Corneal wound burn

Corneal wound burn is less common with modern phaco handpieces and machines.

Incidence
Rare

Onset
Usually evident at the first post-operative visit.

Symptoms
Often none, occasionally foreign-body (gritty) sensation or mild discomfort.

Causes
Thermal injury to the upper lip of the corneal tunnel during phacoemulsification—typically seen after surgery for dense cataracts

Examination findings
Corneal opacification in a semicircular shape at the wound. The surgeon often places a suture if the burn is noted at the end of surgery (see Figure 7.1).

Importance
The shrinkage of corneal tissue may damage the upper lip of the corneal tunnel and may result in early or late (up to a few weeks post-operatively) wound leakage. Wound healing may be delayed and result in excessive astigmatism.

Management
Removal of corneal wound sutures should be delayed for up to 4–6 weeks and performed after discussion with the ophthalmologist.

Descemet detachment

A localized detachment of the Descemet membrane and endothelium. The resulting flap may curl away from the wound.

Incidence
Very rare.

Onset
May be noticed during or at the end of surgery. Small detachments can be left as they settle. Large flaps should be repositioned at the end of surgery with either an air bubble in the anterior chamber or a suture. It may, however, be missed in the presence of corneal oedema following difficult surgery, and it may first be noticed at a post-operative visit.

Symptoms
Glare and blurring of vision from corneal oedema produced by fluid leakage into the corneal stroma.

Causes
Difficult, traumatic or complicated surgery. May also occur if the corneal wound was excessively tight.

Examination findings
There may be an area of localized oedema near the wound. The flap may be seen curled up away from the wound.

Importance
If the flap is large and remains detached for long, it may result in persistent corneal oedema and decompensation.

Management
Small Descemet detachments can be watched and often settle. No action is needed if the corneal clarity is unaffected. If, however, the cornea is oedematous, it may require corrective surgery. Any Descemet detachment should be seen by the ophthalmologist.

Suture irritation

Incidence
Infrequent.

Onset
Any time post-operatively.

Symptoms
Foreign-body sensation.

Causes
May occur if the suture was or has become loose, or if the suture knot is exposed.

Examination findings
The suture may be loose, accumulating mucus. The knot may be visible. The adjoining corneal epithelium may stain with fluorescein.

Importance
It can be a very bothersome symptom and accounts for a significant proportion of unscheduled visits. A loose suture may become a focus for infection.

Management
Loose sutures should be removed, especially after 2 weeks of uncomplicated phacoemulsification cataract surgery and 3 months following routine extracapsular cataract extraction. Suture removal should be considered, particularly if they are accumulating mucus. If the knot is exposed, a bandage contact lens may help until it is safe to remove the suture.

Iris prolapse

Iris prolapse is very rarely seen with modern phacoemulsification techniques.

Incidence
Very rare.

Onset
Typically within the first week.

Symptoms
Pain, foreign-body sensation, watering from the eye.

Causes
Poor wound construction, floppy iris (including patients taking tamsulosin—Flomax), iris trauma during surgery, very rarely partial supra-choroidal haemorrhage.

Examination findings
The iris may reach the inner lip of the wound, or prolapse through it. It will appear as a dark mass at the wound.

Importance
It is a surgical emergency and requires repair.

Management
Needs urgent review by the surgeon for surgical repair (iris repositioning and wound suturing).

Conjunctival chemosis

Incidence
Infrequent.

Onset
Immediately after surgery.

Symptoms
Usually none.

Causes
Leakage of fluid from the phaco probe irrigation sleeve through the wound into the subconjunctival space. Usually seen with a limbal corneal wound placed too posteriorly.

Examination findings
The conjunctiva looks pale and ballooned up all around the limbus.

Importance
Can distort the corneal wound and result in wound leakage.

Management
If the anterior chamber is well formed, no action is needed.
It settles within 1–2 hours.

Hyphaema

Incidence
Very rare.

Onset
May be noticed at the immediate post-operative visit (Figure 8.1).

Symptoms
Blurred vision.

Causes
Leakage from conjunctival vessels at the wound. Rarely due to
bleeding from iris traumatized during surgery.

Examination findings
The blood may be layered or often mixed with fibrin in the
anterior chamber.

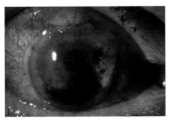

Figure 8.1 Hyphaema seen the next day following a combined phaco-
trabeculectomy and IOL. The hyphaema has arisen either following the
peripheral iridectomy that would have been performed superiorly, or due
to the scleral flap allowing blood to enter the anterior chamber. Note an
iris defect at the 2 o'clock position, near the second corneal incision site,
which occurred due to iris trauma during cataract surgery

Importance
May indicate a leaky wound.

Management
Can be observed if there is no evidence of active bleeding. The Seidel test must be performed to exclude a wound leak and the surgeon should be informed.

Vitreous wick

A vitreous wick is a strand of vitreous coming out of the anterior chamber up to or through the main wound or second incision.

Incidence
Very rare.

Onset
May be noticed at the first or subsequent post-operative visit.

Symptoms
Often none. May present with endophthalmitis or an irritable red eye.

Causes
This can happen after surgery complicated by vitreous loss. However, it may occasionally be seen after uneventful surgery where the vitreous has prolapsed through weak zonules or an unnoticed posterior capsule rupture.

Examination findings
The vitreous strand may be seen reaching up to the wound from the pupillary margin. The pupil may be peaked. The vitreous may be seen on the ocular surface coming through the main wound or second incision.

Importance
It is very important to recognize this complication as it will need prompt referral for surgery. It poses a high risk of

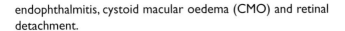

endophthalmitis, cystoid macular oedema (CMO) and retinal detachment.

Management
Prompt referral to the ophthalmologist. Surgery usually involves anterior vitrectomy, however in selected cases YAG laser vitreolysis can be successful in releasing the 'strand' and hence any potential retinal traction.

Corneal-related complications

Mild corneal oedema

Incidence
Common.

Onset
First few days after surgery.

Symptoms
Blurring of vision.

Cause
Endothelial injury from surgical trauma.

Examination findings
Corneal oedema near the wound.

Importance
The severity and duration of oedema correspond to the degree of endothelial trauma.

Management
Observation; resolves without sequelae in the majority of cases. Severe or persistent oedema may need increase in frequency or duration of topical steroid.

Endothelial decompensation (damage) with persistent or severe corneal oedema

Incidence
Very rare.

Onset
May become apparent soon after surgery, but more commonly months to years later.

Symptoms
Blurring of vision worse in the mornings, glare and haloes around lights.

Cause
Poor endothelial reserve, pre-existing endothelial dystrophy, traumatic/complicated surgery, rarely reaction to medications/solutions injected into the anterior chamber during surgery.

Examination findings
Corneal oedema of varying severity.

Importance
Early post-operative endothelial decompensation is serious and may result in a very unfavourable outcome. The surgeon should be informed immediately as it could be due to contaminated fluids used pre-operatively.

Corneal decompensation should prompt a careful look at the fellow eye to look for early signs of endothelial dystrophy that may have been missed pre-operatively.

Management
Mild corneal oedema may settle with topical steroid treatment. Moderate oedema may respond to hypertonic (5%) saline drops. Severe cases may need a corneal graft.

Corneal abrasion

A corneal abrasion may occur in the operated eye or in the fellow eye.

Incidence
Rare.

Onset
Within 24 hours post-operatively.

Symptoms
Pain, scratchy sensation, watering and photophobia.

Cause
In the operated eye, it could be due to accidental injury when removing the speculum at the end of surgery, or trauma from instruments during surgery. It could also be due to the eye remaining open under the eyepad, and sometimes due to excessive handling of tissues, particularly near the wound or second incision.

The fellow eye may develop an abrasion if it was not protected or kept covered when performing surgery under a general anaesthetic. This is, however, very rare.

Examination findings
The abrasion will be evident on fluorescein staining.

Importance
It is an important cause of unscheduled visits post-operatively.

Management
Large abrasions could be patched overnight. Alternatively, lubricant or antibiotic ointment may be instilled 3–4 times a day untill the abrasion heals. Post-operative medications may be safely continued in case of small abrasions, which will heal without intervention.

Uveal complications

Endophthalmitis

Although rare (incidence 1 in 1000), endophthalmitis is one of the most dreaded complications of cataract surgery.

Incidence
Very rare.

Onset
It can present anytime after surgery. Most cases present within the first week. Late onset endophthalmitis is usually due to low-grade organisms and can present a few months later, often manifesting days after the post-operative topical medications are withdrawn.

Symptoms
Redness, pain, watering and reduced vision are the main symptoms. Symptoms usually come on over 24–48 hours. Pain is an ominous symptom and should prompt urgent referral.

Cause
Usually entry of organisms into the anterior chamber during surgery. The usual organisms are from the periocular skin and eyelid flora. Rarely may be due to a leaky wound or vitreous wick introducing infection post-operatively. Complicated and prolonged surgery increases the risk.

Examination findings
Reduced visual acuity, often down to hand movements or count fingers. There may be fibrin in the anterior chamber, hypopyon and a hazy (Figure 8.2) or no view of the posterior segment.

Importance
It is one of the few true surgical emergencies. Urgent action is essential.

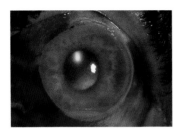

Figure 8.2 Early post-operative endophthalmitis within 3 days of surgery. There is a hypopyon in the anterior chamber and a very hazy view of the posterior segment, and the patient's vision was reduced to 2/60

Management

Vitreous biopsy and intravitreal antibiotic injection must be performed urgently (within hours) to prevent irreversible damage to the eye and vision. Hospital admission and prolonged treatment with topical and systemic antibiotics as well as steroids are usually needed. Recovery is slow and often incomplete.

Persistent uveitis

Incidence
Infrequent.

Onset
Some degree of anterior chamber activity (anterior chamber inflammation signified by cells and flare) is expected after uncomplicated cataract surgery. This may persist longer if surgery was complicated, but rarely beyond 3–4 weeks. Topical steroid treatment is usually discontinued at one-month. Occasionally, the uveitis may persist for longer, and the eye will flare up within days of discontinuing the topical treatment—this is termed persistent uveitis. Rarely, the uveitis may return weeks after discontinuing treatment and is termed recurrent uveitis.

Symptoms
Often asymptomatic. In more severe cases, symptoms include redness, photophobia, pain, watering and blurred vision.

Cause

Persistent uveitis may be due to retained lens matter, particularly in the capsular bag or sulcus, although this may not be readily visible despite fully dilating the pupil. It may also be due to early discontinuation of steroid treatment and individual variation in response to surgery. Uveitis persists longer in diabetics, in eyes with dark coloured irides and following complicated surgery. Very rarely, it may be a sign of low-grade endophthalmitis or may be seen in association with CMO.

Examination findings

Circum-corneal injection, 1+ or more cells in the anterior chamber and flare.

Importance

It is important to recognize persistent anterior chamber activity so that treatment may be continued for longer.

Management

Continuation of steroid treatment for longer.

Recurrent uveitis

Incidence

Rare.

Onset

Rarely, the uveitis may return weeks after discontinuing treatment.

Symptoms

Redness, photophobia, pain, watering and blurred vision.

Cause

Recurrent uveitis may be due to retained lens matter, particularly in the capsular bag or sulcus. A malpositioned IOL (especially if one or both of the haptics are in the sulcus) may irritate the ciliary body and produce low-grade uveitis. Very rarely, it may be a sign of low-grade endophthalmitis, or seen in association with CMO.

Examination findings
Circum-corneal injection, 1+ or more cells in the anterior chamber and flare.

Importance
It is important to perform a thorough dilated examination to look for capsular deposits (seen in low-grade bacterial endophthalmitis) or retained lens matter. Vitreous activity is not expected after post-cataract uveitis and would suggest the possibility of endophthalmitis. The position of the IOL must be assessed to exclude a malpositioned IOL as a cause.

Management
Most cases will respond to a course of topical steroid. Resistant or persistent cases may indicate the need for definitive treatment of the cause if found. A malpositioned IOL may have to be repositioned or exchanged. Retained lens matter may need to be removed. Low-grade endophthalmitis may respond to intravitreal antibiotic injection.

Iris defects

Incidence
Very rare.

Onset
Symptoms from iris trauma will be evident within days of surgery.

Symptoms
Monocular diplopia and glare from excess light entering the eye.

Cause
Trauma during surgery.

Examination findings
There may be a defect in the iris at the pupillary margin, or more commonly in the periphery near the side port (produced by iris chafing) (Figure 8.1 and Figure 8.3).

Importance
Patients may be very symptomatic with larger defects.

Management
The symptoms often settle with time. Persistent symptoms may need a dark coloured contact lens with a central clear pupil, or surgical repair.

Lens-related complications

IOL decentration
Incidence
Very rare.

Onset
May develop soon after surgery if capsular support was compromised during surgery. Late decentration can occur several months or years later.

Symptoms
Blurred vision, glare from the edge effect and monocular diplopia.

Figure 8.3 Iris trauma during complicated cataract surgery

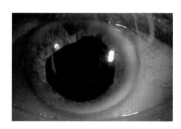

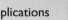
Cause
May be due to lack of capsular support or zonular dehiscence. It can also occur as a result of asymmetric contraction of the capsular bag.

Examination findings
The edge of the lens may be visible in the pupillary area in mild to moderate cases of decentration. In severe cases, the entire optic may be displaced out of the visual axis, or even dislocated into the anterior chamber or vitreous cavity (Figure 8.4).

Importance
Decentred IOLs can produce annoying symptoms and may require corrective surgery.

Management
Observation in mild cases. IOL repositioning or exchange in severe cases.

IOL haptic prolapse

Incidence
Very rare.

Onset
Usually evident within a day or two of surgery, if not at the immediate post-operative check.

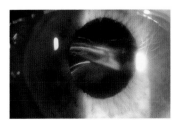

Figure 8.4 IOL decentration due to compromised zonular capsule support following complicated cataract surgery (Courtesy of Anne Bolton, Oxford Eye Hospital)

Symptoms

Foreign-body sensation, irritable red eye. Sometimes asymptomatic and detected at the post-operative check.

Cause

Incomplete insertion of IOL.

Examination findings

One of the IOL haptics may be in front of the iris (Figure 8.5), resulting in a peaked pupil. Rarely, the haptic may be in the wound, or even protruding through the wound.

Importance

This complication requires surgical correction and hence prompt referral.

Management

Surgical repositioning of the IOL.

Posterior capsular opacification

Posterior capsular opacification (PCO) is one of the commonest complications of cataract surgery. It affects 25–50% of patients 2 years after surgery.

Incidence

Common.

Figure 8.5 IOL haptic prolapse in front of the iris (Courtesy of Anne Bolton, Oxford Eye Hospital)

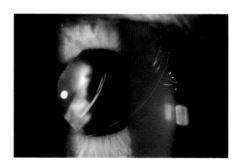

Onset

Typically develops over months or years after surgery. It can happen within weeks to months in some cases, particularly younger patients.

Symptoms

Patients describe hazy or misty vision. Glare may be an associated symptom.

Cause

Residual lens epithelial cells are inevitably left behind at the time of surgery, attached to the capsule despite meticulous removal of soft lens matter. They proliferate, migrate and undergo metaplasia, resulting in opacification of the posterior capsule. Two patterns of posterior capsular opacification are seen: cellular proliferation, producing drop-like deposits in the visual axis (Elschnig's pearls), or fibrosis and shrinkage of the capsule, producing striae.

Examination findings

Elschnig's pearls are large droplet-like deposits on the posterior capsule (Figure 8.6). There may be striae and a fibrous sheet across the visual axis.

Importance

PCO develops gradually in most cases. As a result, patients may not be aware of the gradual but often significant reduction in vision. Many cases would see their optometrist for a change of

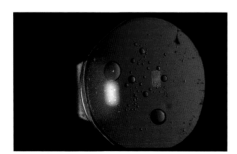

Figure 8.6 Late PCO following cataract surgery. Elschnig's pearls are visible as large droplet-like deposits on the posterior capsule (Courtesy of Anne Bolton, Oxford Eye Hospital)

glasses, who would detect PCO and refer them to the ophthalmologist for treatment.

Management

There is now considerable evidence that square-profile IOLs reduce the risk of PCO. The emphasis has shifted from treatment to prevention of PCO as our understanding of the condition has improved.

YAG laser capsulotomy is a very effective and safe procedure for the treatment of visually significant PCO. It is performed as an outpatient procedure and does not require any anaesthesia.

Retained lens matter

Retained matter may be soft lens (cortex) or hard (nucleus).

Incidence
Rare.

Onset
Retained nuclear fragments or soft lens matter may be visible in the anterior chamber at the first or subsequent post-operative visit. However, the presentation is sometimes delayed.

Symptoms
Blurred vision from fluffy lens matter in the visual axis or corneal oedema produced by nuclear remnants. Photophobia and redness may be due to excessive or persistent uveitis.

Cause
Complicated surgery or intraoperative miosis may result in incomplete 'cortical clean up'. Nuclear fragments may remain hidden in the ciliary sulcus or the anterior chamber angle.

Examination findings
Fluffy soft lens matter may be visible in the capsular bag or anterior chamber. Nuclear fragments may be visible in the angle of the anterior chamber. However, they are not always readily

seen and may be simply manifest by localized corneal oedema or
persistent uveitis.

Importance
Retained lens matter may produce a brisk uveitis, CMO and
corneal changes that can affect vision. If left untreated, it may
become organized into a dense sheet over the posterior capsule,
which may be difficult to treat with the YAG laser.

Management
Most cases will respond to a prolonged course of topical steroid.
Small to moderate amounts of retained soft lens matter will
resorb in most cases, especially if it is anterior to the IOL. Larger
amounts that persist may have to be removed surgically if they
obscure the visual axis or produce significant uveitis.

Phimosis (constriction) of anterior capsule

Incidence
Very rare.

Onset
Usually occurs months to years after surgery.

Symptoms
Often asymptomatic. Extreme phimosis may produce darkening of
the image by significantly reducing the light entering the eye, or
may even completely obscure the visual axis.

Cause
It is believed to be caused by fibrotic reaction of the anterior
capsule stimulated by residual lens epithelial cells on its
undersurface. The risk is increased if the capsulorrhexis is small.

Examination findings
The anterior capsular opening is reduced, and may be pinpoint in
extreme cases. There is considerable stretch on the zonules as a
result.

Importance

Severe phimosis requires surgical correction. It is particularly relevant in diabetics, who are more prone to develop phimosis, and will need a detailed fundus examination for assessing and treating diabetic retinopathy.

Management

Surgical anterior capsulotomy. YAG laser capsulotomy may be attempted in mild to moderate cases to produce relaxing radial openings in the constricting band.

Refractive complications

Ametropia

Ametropia is an unexpected refractive result where the spherical refractive error is greater than expected or is outside what the patient or surgeon would consider acceptable.

Incidence

Common.

Onset

May become evident as soon as any corneal and wound oedema and uveitis resolve and the vision starts to clear. This could be within a few days of surgery, although some patients may not report it until their scheduled post-operative visit.

Symptoms

Poor unaided vision. Vision may improve by screwing the eyes up, thereby obtaining a pinhole effect.

Cause

Typically caused by biometry errors, or less commonly by wrong choice of IOL power. Very rarely mislabelling of IOL power (manufacturing error).

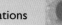
Examination findings
Poor unaided visual acuity, improves considerably with pinhole or refraction.

Importance
It is important to recognize this complication early so that remedial action, such as lens exchange, can be offered.

Management
Depends on the degree of ametropia and the requirements and expectations of the patient. The tolerance level for post-operative ametropia varies from patient to patient, and also between surgeons. Some patients would accept up to 2 D or even 3 D of ametropia, whereas others may be dissatisfied with greater than 1 D. It is important to remember that unaided vision drops to 6/18 and 6/36 with 1 D and 2 D of spherical error, respectively. Most cases can be managed with appropriate spectacle correction if the anisometropia is not intolerable (generally under 3 D). Contact lens correction, LASIK, implantable contact lenses, piggyback IOLs and lens exchange are other means of correcting anisometropia. The surgeon will discuss the various options, including the risks and benefits of each, with the patient.

Induced astigmatism

Some degree of astigmatism is expected after cataract surgery. Although much lower with phacoemulsification compared with extracapsular surgery, excessive astigmatism still remains a significant cause of poor uncorrected vision after cataract surgery.

Incidence
Common.

Onset
May become evident as soon as any corneal and wound oedema or uveitis resolve and the vision begins to improve. This could be

within a few days of surgery, although some patients may not report it until their scheduled post-operative visit, or indeed not at all.

Symptoms
Poor uncorrected visual acuity.

Cause
Poorly constructed or large wounds or wound distortion from corneal wound burn or sutures. Wound slippage is more common after superior than temporal incisions and can produce gradual against-the-rule astigmatism.

Examination findings
Poor uncorrected vision.

Importance
It is a correctable cause of poor acuity. Excessive astigmatism may need referral to the ophthalmologist for consideration of removal of tight corneal sutures or even refractive surgery.

Management
Pre-existing astigmatism may be dealt with (reduced or corrected) at the time of surgery with correct placement of incision, with or without paired phaco incisions or limbal relaxing incisions.

Optical correction with glasses or toric contact lenses is usually adequate in the majority of cases of induced or residual astigmatism. Excess induced astigmatism may be an indication for refractive surgery (implantable contact lens, LASIK or arcuate keratotomy). Tight corneal sutures along the same meridian as the steepest corneal curvature should obviously be removed before final spectacles are prescribed.

Glare from lens-edge effect with square-profile IOLs

Incidence
Rare.

Onset
May become evident as soon as any corneal and wound oedema and uveitis resolve and the vision starts to clear. This could be within a few days of surgery, although some patients may not report it until their scheduled post-operative visit, or even months after surgery.

Symptoms
Dazzle and glare, especially with artificial lights, obliquely placed light sources, and oncoming headlights when driving.

Cause
The square edge of some of the modern IOLs can reflect light internally, producing glare.

Examination findings
No significant abnormality will be found. Diagnosis is based on knowledge of the IOL chosen.

Importance
This symptom can be very annoying. Recognition of the cause and adequate explanation are often the key to resolving patient anxieties.

Management
This issue has been addressed with most new-generation IOLs. Frosted square edges, for example, do not permit internal reflection. Most cases settle spontaneously as the peripheral anterior capsule opacifies. Rarely, sunglasses, clear pupil painted contact lenses or even topical medication to constrict the pupil (for example Brimonidine or even dilute Pilocarpine) have been required.

Posterior segment complications

Cystoid macular oedema

Incidence
Infrequent; the incidence of transient CMO is approximately 2% at 4–6 weeks after surgery.

Onset
First 4–6 weeks after surgery.

Symptoms
Deterioration in vision occurring after a period of improved acuity. Some patients may describe slight redness and discomfort or photophobia.

Cause
Often idiopathic. Rarely secondary to retinal vein occlusion or epiretinal membrane. More common after complicated cataract surgery, particularly vitreous loss. Other risk factors include retained lens matter and irritation of the iris or ciliary body by a malpositioned posterior chamber IOL or anterior chamber IOL. Pre-existing uveitis and diabetes are other risk factors. Elevated levels of intraocular prostaglandins are believed to play a role.

Examination findings
Reduced corrected visual acuity. There may be 1+ or 2+ cells in the anterior chamber or vitreous. The macular reflex may be dulled, and in advanced cases there may be haemorrhages or even intraretinal cysts.

Importance
CMO is a relatively common cause of an unfavourable outcome of otherwise uneventful surgery.

Management
Fluorescein angiography used to be the diagnostic test of choice before the advent of optical coherence tomography (OCT), a non-invasive test that provides cross-sectional images through the macula. OCT can aid measurement of macular thickness, demonstrate cystic changes and monitor improvement.

Mild CMO may resolve without any treatment. Most ophthalmologists would, however, treat with a combination of topical steroid, e.g. dexamethasone 0.1%, and non-steroid anti-inflammatory medication, e.g. ketorolac four times a day. Treatment may have to be continued for up to 3 months. Some

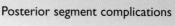
cases may respond initially only to return as treatment is withdrawn. Resistant cases may respond to sub-Tenon's or intravitreal injection of steroid. Some cases may not respond and may result in a poor visual outcome.

Posterior vitreous detachment

Incidence
Common.

Onset
Posterior vitreous detachment (PVD) can occur days, weeks or even months after surgery.

Symptoms
Flashes and floaters, blurring of vision.

Cause
The process of removing the crystalline lens from the eye and replacing it with a much thinner IOL creates a dead space. As a result, the vitreous moves forward, which may precipitate detachment from the posterior pole.

Examination findings
Opacities may be seen in the vitreous, including a Weiss' ring, a ring-shaped vitreous condensation floating anterior to the optic disc (Figure 8.7). It is important to look for pigmented or blood cells in the vitreous cavity ("tobacco dust").

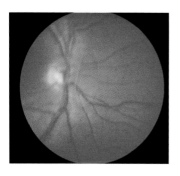

Figure 8.7 A Weiss' ring floating anterior to the optic disc, indicating a PVD

Importance
PVD could be accompanied by a retinal tear or haemorrhage.

Management
A detailed dilated fundus examination is mandatory. If no retinal pathology is found, the patient can be reassured, with a full explanation.

Retinal tear or detachment

Incidence
Very rare; incidence of retinal detachment is 1 in 1000 after cataract surgery. The risk is greater in myopic eyes.

Onset
Can occur within days of surgery, or months or even years later.

Symptoms
Symptoms of PVD along with blurring of vision. Field defect may be reported if the detachment extends towards the posterior pole.

Cause
The retina is usually pulled off at the site of abnormal vitreo-retinal adhesion during the separation of the posterior vitreous.

Examination findings
Usually a U-shaped peripheral retinal tear with some vitreous debris. Examination by direct ophthalmoscopy is **not** sufficient to locate a peripheral retinal tear. A dilated fundus examination with indirect slit-lamp biomicroscopy is required at a minimum. It is useful to note that the presence of brown pigmented cells ('tobacco dust') and blood cells in the anterior vitreous are highly suggestive of the presence of a retinal tear. Sometimes the vitreous may pull off an operculum, resulting in a round hole.

Importance
If not detected and treated, it could progress to retinal detachment and loss of vision.

Management
U-shaped tears have manifest traction and need treating. Round holes have no ongoing traction and can be left untreated as there is a very low risk of detachment.

Posterior tears can be treated with argon laser surround. Peripheral tears may need cryotherapy treatment.

Closed suprachoroidal haemorrhage

Incidence
Very rare.

Onset
Can occur per-operatively but remain undetected until the post-operative check. However, can also occur hours or even days after surgery.

Symptoms
Severe pain is the hallmark of suprachoroidal haemorrhage. Depending on the extent of the haemorrhage, the vision may or may not be affected.

Cause
Spontaneous rupture of choroidal vessels. Risk factors include dense black or brown cataracts, systemic hypertension, obesity and surgery complicated by vitreous loss.

Examination findings
Shallow or flat anterior chamber, hyphaema, iris prolapse, high intraocular pressure (IOP) and a dark subretinal mass in the periphery extending centrally. It may also occur as a complication of hypotony in association with choroidal effusions (Figure 8.8).

Importance
Needs urgent referral as it could potentially result in complete loss of vision, or even loss of the eye as a result of an expulsive haemorrhage if the wound is not secure.

Figure 8.8
Suprachoroidal haemorrhage: occurred as a complication of hypotony due to persistent wound leak following cataract surgery (Courtesy of C. K. Patel)

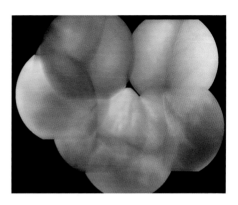

Management
Usually conservative. IOP must be lowered, and wound integrity restored if not secure. May need surgical evacuation of suprachoroidal blood in some cases.

Progression of coexistent retinal disease

Coexistent retinal diseases include diabetic retinopathy and age-related macular degeneration (ARMD).

Incidence
Infrequent.

Onset
Within weeks to months of cataract surgery.

Symptoms
Deterioration in vision after initial improvement.

Cause
Prostaglandin release as part of the post-operative inflammation is believed to play a role.

Examination findings
Changes of diabetic maculopathy (exudates or macular oedema) or wet ARMD may be seen.

Importance
Patients with coexistent retinal disease should be examined carefully post-operatively and more frequently with dilated fundus examinations. The first dilated examination should be within 1 month of surgery.

Management
Laser treatment or intravitreal steroid injection for diabetic maculopathy. Fluorescein angiography and further treatment based thereon in cases with macular degeneration.

Glaucoma

Post-operative raised intraocular pressure

Incidence
Common.

Onset
A significant proportion of patients undergoing cataract surgery will develop transient rise in IOP post-operatively. The maximum elevation occurs within the first 24 hours, and usually within the first few hours after surgery. It drops sharply thereafter. The mean rise in IOP is 8–10 mmHg, and over 30 mmHg in fewer than 2% of patients. Furthermore, fewer than 2% of patients will have a raised IOP after 24 hours. The incidence and IOP levels are much higher after complicated surgery.

Symptoms
Pain, and misty vision if the pressure is very high. Often asymptomatic.

Cause
Overinflation of the anterior chamber at the end of surgery and obstruction of the aqueous outflow system with retained viscoelastic (for example, Healon) used during surgery are

common causes. Prolonged and traumatic surgery is more likely to produce raised pressure.

Examination findings

Corneal oedema may be evident, particularly with very high pressures (over 40 mmHg). Residual viscoelastic may be visible in the anterior chamber in addition to possible blood and fibrin in some cases. The anterior chamber may be excessively deep. If the anterior chamber is shallow and pressure raised, it is important to look for a partial suprachoroidal haemorrhage.

Importance

Glaucoma patients with damaged discs are particularly vulnerable to further damage as a result of post-operative spikes of IOP. There is a risk of developing vascular occlusions, for example central retinal vein or artery occlusion, or anterior ischaemic optic neuropathy. Persistent raised pressure beyond 48 hours should raise suspicion of retained viscoelastic or lens matter.

Management

Some surgeons routinely use acetazolamide (Diamox) post-operatively to prevent rise in IOP. Transient elevated pressures of up to 30 mmHg can be monitored and usually settle without problems. Higher pressures may need treatment with oral acetazolamide or topical pressure-lowering drops. Very high IOP may be treated with release of aqueous from the side incision, particularly if the anterior chamber is excessively deep.

Steroid-induced glaucoma

Incidence

Rare.

Onset

Usually occurs a few days or weeks after surgery.

Symptoms

Usually none.

Cause

Up to a third of the population will demonstrate a rise in IOP in response to topical or systemic steroid treatment ('steroid responders') for no apparent reason. It is believed to be due to deposition of material in the trabecular meshwork. This is a consistent and repeatable pattern for every episode of steroid treatment in that individual.

Examination findings

Raised IOP.

Importance

It is important to check the IOP at the final post-operative visit as the pressure can sometimes reach a dangerously high level. It is also important to document steroid responsiveness in the records and make the patient and doctors (ophthalmologist and GP) aware as the patient may need steroid treatment in the future for unrelated reasons.

Management

The IOP rise is usually transient and responds to withdrawal of steroid treatment and topical IOP-lowering agents. If, however, prolonged steroid treatment becomes necessary, regular monitoring and treatment of IOP is essential.

Eyelid-related complications

Ptosis

Incidence

Very rare.

Onset

Usually noted a few months after surgery.

Symptoms

Patients report a droopy upper eyelid on the operated side.

Cause

Ptosis occurring after cataract surgery is poorly understood. More often seen following extracapsular surgery, it was believed to be due to localized levator atrophy produced by a haematoma during placement of the superior rectus bridle suture. It has also been suggested that excessive stretching of the eyelid skin on peeling away the surgical drape may also play a role in disinsertion of the levator aponeurosis.

Examination findings

Mild ptosis with good levator function.

Importance

Elderly patients may have a degree of pre-existing ptosis due to levator dehiscence. The small eyelid droop produced may be sufficient to drop the eyelid further and affect vision.

Management

Ptosis correction may be indicated. It may be advisable to delay surgery until after the contralateral eye has undergone cataract surgery as the other side may develop ptosis.

Drug-related allergy or adverse effects

Preservative or drug allergy

Incidence

Infrequent.

Onset

Usually evident within a few days of starting topical medications. The allergy may be either to the specific drug or to the preservative.

Symptoms

Redness, irritation, watering and stinging sensation on instilling drops.

Cause
Poorly understood, but believed to be due to an idiosyncratic reaction.

Examination findings
Conjunctival injection often more marked in the inferior fornix, punctuate corneal staining, eyelid oedema and erythema may be present.

Importance
Some patients may discontinue post-operative medications prematurely if they cause discomfort. Early cessation of medication may result in persistence or flare-up of post-operative uveitis.

Management
If preservative allergy is suspected (more common than drug allergy) then switch to preservative-free preparations. True allergy to steroids is extremely rare and may benefit from substitution with non-steroidal agents, such as ketorolac. If antibiotic allergy is suspected, the usual antibiotic–steroid combination can be substituted with a steroid-only preparation. Antibiotics are usually not required once the wound edge has epithelialized (within 1 week).

Acetozolamide adverse effects

Incidence
Common; adverse effects due to acetozolamide are surprisingly common.

Onset
Can manifest within 12–24 hours.

Symptoms
Tingling numbness (paraesthesia), metallic taste, nausea, excessive tiredness and malaise.

Cause
Potassium depletion.

Examination findings
Nil.

Importance
Usually short-lasting symptoms, but can be very distressing for some patients.

Management
Plenty of fluids. Recommend intake of citrus fruits and juices. Discontinuation of medication.

Extraocular movements

Diplopia

Incidence
Very rare.

Onset
Patients may report diplopia for a few hours after surgery under local anaesthesia as the operated eye may not have recovered its full range of movement. Diplopia can also occur months or even years later, and is often vertical.

Symptoms
Some patients may report two distinct images, others may describe ghosting or blurring of images. The separation of the images is often vertical.

Cause
It may be seen following surgery under peribulbar or sub-Tenon's anaesthesia. It is believed to be due to fibrosis in or around the inferior rectus or oblique muscles following bleeding due to anaesthetic injection.

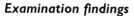
Examination findings
Usually a small vertical deviation but with a nearly full range of eye movements. Plotting the range of eye movements with the Hess chart is useful. A full orthoptic assessment is necessary in most cases.

Importance
The vertical fusion range is usually quite small, and even a small separation of images can produce bothersome symptoms which the patient cannot overcome. The occurrence of the complication may influence the choice of anaesthetic for surgery on the fellow eye.

Management
Prisms are often helpful. Fresnel prisms may be tried initially before incorporation into glasses.

Conclusion

Most complications are thankfully rare and minor. Furthermore, the majority of these complications may not be sight-threatening. However, it is important to recognize the more serious complications and refer urgently to ensure a favourable outcome.

Further reading

Barak, A., Desatnik, H., Ma-Naim, T., Ashkenasi, I., Neufeld, A. and Melamed, S. (1996). Early postoperative intraocular pressure pattern in glaucomatous and nonglaucomatous patients. *J. Cataract. Refract. Surg.* **22**(5): 607–611.

Dewey, S. (2006). Posterior capsule opacification. *Curr. Opin. Ophthalmol.* **17**(1): 45–53.

Hayashi, K. and Hayashi, H. (2005). Posterior capsule opacification in the presence of an intraocular lens with a sharp versus rounded optic edge. *Ophthalmology* **112**(9): 1550–1556.

Jonas, J.B., Kreissig, I. and Degenring, R.F. (2003). Intravitreal triamcinolone acetonide for pseudophakic cystoid macular edema. *Am. J. Ophthalmol.* **136**(2): 384–386.

Singal, N. and Hopkins, J.. Pseudophakic cystoid macular edema: ketorolac alone vs. ketorolac plus prednisolone. *Can. J. Ophthalmol.* **39**(3): 245–250.

Sunaric-Megevand, G. and Pournaras, C.J. (1997). Current approach to postoperative endophthalmitis. *Br. J. Ophthalmol.* **81**(11): 1006–1015.

Tan, J.H., Newman, D.K., Klunker, C., Watts, S.E. and Burton, R.L. (2000). Phacoemulsification cataract surgery: is routine review necessary on the first post-operative day? *Eye* **14**(1): 53–55.

Thirumalai, B. and Baranyovits, P.R. (2003). Intraocular pressure changes and the implications on patient review after phacoemulsification. *J. Cataract. Refract. Surg.* **29**(3): 504–507.

Tuft, S.J., Minassian, D. and Sullivan, P. (2006). Risk factors for retinal detachment after cataract surgery: a case-control study. *Ophthalmology* **113**(4): 650–656.

9

Paediatric cataract: aetiology, diagnosis and management

Samer Hamada

Introduction

Congenital cataract requires urgent attention; early treatment is the factor that most determines the final visual outcome. Visual development and maturation can be severely affected by the presence of lens opacities during the first ten years of life. The earlier these opacities occur and the denser they are, the less likely it is that the child will develop good vision.

Although the visual prognosis for monocular congenital cataract is worse than that for bilateral congenital cataracts due to severe amblyopia, the latter still accounts for a significant number of children being registered as legally blind each year. Early detection of cataract can be simple, by performing the red reflex examination in the newly born child. Occasionally, the cataract can be difficult to detect, manifesting at a later age when it affects the child's visual functions.

Surgical and optical treatment may not help in achieving useful vision, particularly in monocular cases.

Aetiology of paediatric cataract

It is important to remember that paediatric cataract is not always an isolated disease. It can be part of metabolic disorders or genetically transmitted syndromes. The aetiology can be difficult to diagnose. Interestingly, the majority of these cataracts are idiopathic (60–80%).

Bilateral cataracts are usually inherited (up to 70% of cases). The most common type of inheritance is autosomal dominant. Bilateral nuclear opacities are the most common autosomal dominant inherited form of cataract. These cataracts may be

Congenital cataract requires **urgent attention**. Early detection and treatment are the most important factors that determine the final visual outcomes.

isolated (30%), associated with ocular manifestations (2%) such as aniridia, microphthalmus and anterior segment dysgenesis, or may be associated with systemic, metabolic and genetic disorders (5%) such as Hallerman–Streiff and Lowe's syndromes, galactosemia and craniofacial abnormalities. Intrauterine infections are the cause in 3% of cases, usually resulting in dense, central and bilateral cataracts.

Unilateral cataract, however, is rarely associated with systemic or genetic disease. It may occur in association with other ocular abnormalities (10%), such as posterior lenticonus, persistent hyperplastic primary vitreous (PHPV) and anterior segment dysgenesis. Eye trauma accounts for 10% of unilateral cataracts. In contrast to bilateral cataracts, intrauterine infections are unlikely to cause unilateral cataract (however, it may rarely be due to rubella infection). Child abuse must be excluded in paediatric traumatic cataracts.

Cataract morphology

It is important to emphasize that paediatric cataracts can have a wide spectrum of presentations and variations, which in turn affect prognosis.

The morphological type of paediatric cataract helps to predict the aetiology, the age of onset and the visual prognosis and it sometimes suggests heritability. It is essential to document the location and morphological characteristics of any cataract, particularly in congenital cases. This often helps identify age of onset in addition to aetiology.

Some cataracts hardly progress, for example anterior polar and nuclear cataracts. However, the more common cataracts

> Bilateral cataracts are usually inherited (mostly as autosomal dominant), in contrast to unilateral cataract, which usually occurs as an isolated case.

such as lamellar and PHPV can continue to progress throughout life.

Clinical diagnosis

Paediatric cataract should be considered as a systemic disease and management should be approached with this in mind. The clinical diagnosis and management plan should be based on the following assessments:

A. History
B. Ocular examination
C. Systemic examination
D. Investigations
E. Genetic and paediatric consultations.

A. History

a. Age of onset
b. Symptoms (if any)
c. Childhood medical history, including previous trauma (mainly in unilateral cataract)
d. Family history (particularly in bilateral cataracts)
e. General development (developmental delay is associated with bilateral cataract).

B. Ocular examination

a. Observation: ocular examination of infants and young children can be challenging. Nevertheless, a lot of the information can be obtained from observing the child's visual behaviour and the alignment of both eyes. The presence of strabismus can indicate the development of amblyopia in the deviated eye. Photophobia or a disoriented child may be the only signs of cataract.
b. Red reflex test: simple and helpful for all ages, but most importantly for those up to 6 months of age. It is usually performed by a paediatrician, general practitioner or a nurse.

Dilated ocular examination using a direct ophthalmoscope or retinoscope is essential to perform this test (Figure 9.1, Figure 9.2). The red reflex test can be of great value in answering the following questions:

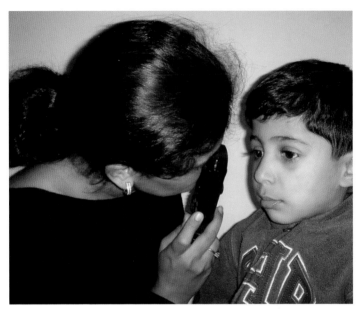

Figure 9.1 Direct ophthalmoscope is useful for looking at the retinal red reflex, thus identifying any lens opacity. More detail of the lens opacity can be seen by using a +5 D lens in the ophthalmoscope

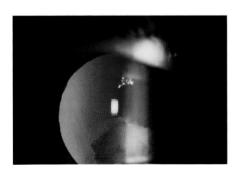

Figure 9.2 Red reflex showing inferior lens opacity

1. Is the cataract unilateral or bilateral?
2. Is the cataract central?
3. How dense is the cataract and is it obscuring fundus view?

c. **Visual assessment**: one of the key determenants when making a decision of whether to operate or not. Understanding the visual behaviour and methods to measure the vision for each age group is essential in assessing a child with cataract. Steady fixation dose not occur before 6 weeks of age. By 8 weeks the child starts to follow objects. Visual acuity at birth can be less than 6/60 and then develops gradually. Recognition visual acuity of 6/6 might not be achieved until age 7 (Snellen acuity). Visual evoked potential (VEP) can be used at any age, particularly if there is difficulty in measuring the child's ability to see or if visual pathway disease is suspected.

1. **Neonates**: the ability of the child to fixate develops after 6–8 weeks of age. Therefore, the red reflex test and clinical examination are the only reliable methods to decide whether the cataract is visually significant or not. Central cataracts that measure more than 3 mm, posterior cataracts, and total cataracts that obscure fundus view are usually visually significant. Polar and sutural cataracts, though central, have minimal visual effects.

2. **Children age 3–18 months**: the simplest way to check vision in this age group is to test whether fixation is central or eccentric. When performing the fixation test, the examiner should be able to document whether the fixation is central, steady and maintained (often referred to as the CSM system). This test can be performed in monocular and binocular testing (Figure 9.3). A vertical 10 D prism can also be used to dissociate the eyes (Figure 9.4).

   Standard fixation preference testing can diagnose moderate to severe amblyopia in patients with tropias greater than 10 prism dioptre (PD). Patients with small-angle deviations or straight eyes should be examined with the 10-Δ fixation test, with the criterion for equal vision being the ability to hold fixation well, with either eye through smooth pursuit.

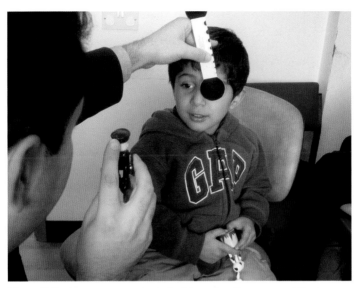

Figure 9.3 Cover test to check for binocular alignment and fixation preference

Objection to occlusion indicates the presence of amblyopia (Figure 9.5). However, bilateral cataract can result in bilateral amblyopia, which is difficult to show with an occlusion test. It is important to differentiate between the child's fears of the examiner's approach and the presence of amblyopia. Preferential-looking tests, such as Teller and Keeler acuity cards and the Cardiff Acuity Test (Figure 9.6), are useful, especially when comparing the two eyes of a child. As some of these tests rely on ocular movement for objective measure, children with ocular motor disease might give a negative response to such tests, thus giving rise to false negatives.

3. **Children older than 2 years**: it becomes easier to measure the visual acuity in this age group. Kay pictures (Figure 9.7), Sheridan–Gardiner plates, single letters and Snellen acuity charts measure a child's recognition acuity.

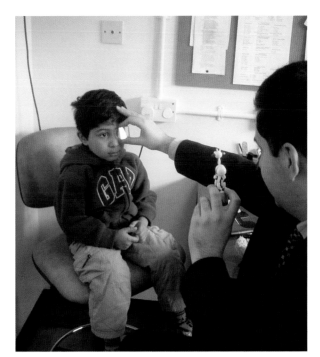

Figure 9.4   A 10 D vertical prism (base down here) is generally used to detect fixation in children and infants with no strabismus. The expected normal response is that the eye without prism will take over fixation. Fixation with the eye that is under prism suggests a visual problem in the other eye

- Not all types of cataract are visually significant.
- Infants do not normally fixate before 6 weeks of age.
- Observation, red reflex test and clinical examination are the main sources of information to predict the level of vision in children less than 6 weeks of age.
- The CSM system is an important test to check fixation in children above 3 months of age.

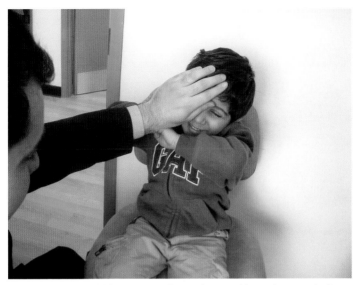

Figure 9.5   The child objects to the occlusion of his right eye, which indicates moderate-to-severe amblyopia in his left eye

d. Comprehensive ocular examination: this should include:
1. Ocular motor examination to reveal any strabismus, which should be performed for both near and distant fixation. Abnormal head posture can often be noticed during this test, and attention should be made to correct this while performing the test (Figure 9.8).
2. Testing for stereopsis, a function of binocular vision. Lang, TNO, Titmus Fly and Frisby tests can be used to quantitatively assess the stereoacuity of a child (Figure 9.9).
3. Pupil reflexes, to exclude the presence of a relative afferent pupillary defect suggestive of an anterior visual pathway disorder.
4. Slit lamp examination; a handheld slit lamp is an essential tool for examining infants and uncooperative children.
5. A systematic ocular examination, including eyelids, conjunctiva, cornea, lens and anterior and posterior segments.

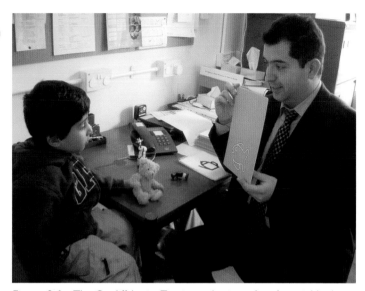

Figure 9.6 The Cardiff Acuity Test is a selection of preferential looking pictures designed to measure acuity in toddlers aged 1–3 years and in individuals with intellectual impairment. It combines the principles of preferential looking and vanishing optotypes. Note how the child fixates on the picture

6. Intraocular pressure, which should be checked prior to any surgical intervention, either by Perkins tonometry or a tonopen.

Certain clinical findings may allude to the diagnosis; for example, the presence of a cloudy cornea in anterior segment dysgenesis, pseudopolycoria (multiple pupils) in Reiger's syndrome, and signs of ocular trauma in child abuse (ocular haemorrhages).

C. Systemic examination

a. **Systemic disease**: presence of clinical signs.
b. **Skeletal abnormalities**: particularly of typical morphological syndromic features.

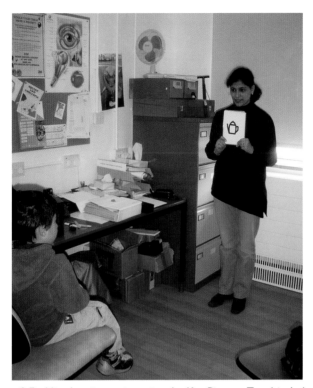

Figure 9.7 Visual acuity testing using the Kay Pictures Test (singles).
Remember that the amblyopic eye performs better with single letter
acuity testing, therefore it is advisable to use a crowded Kay book
whenever possible despite being difficult to use with younger children

The principles of ocular examination of paediatric cataract include:

- visual assessment and presence of amblyopia
- location and morphology of the cataract
- presence of other lens abnormalities (subluxation, PHPV)
- presence of anterior segment dysgenesis (e.g. iris hypoplasia and
  posterior embryotoxon)
- other ocular findings
- ocular ultrasound if there is no view of the fundus
- examination of family members in case of bilateral cataracts.

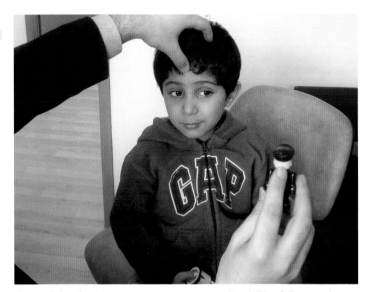

Figure 9.8 Ocular movement examination: the child is following the target, which requires normal saccadic eye movement

D. Investigations

In general, unilateral cataract requires less extensive investigation in comparison to bilateral cataract. However, in a healthy child with bilateral cataracts and a positive family history of autosomal dominant inheritance cataracts, there is usually no need for extensive investigations.

a. **Serum TORCHS titre screen** (TOxoplasmosis, Rubella, Cytomegalic inclusion disease, Herpes simplex and Syphilis).
b. **VDRL titre**: a blood test for syphilis antibodies in the bloodstream.
c. **Urine**: test for reducing substances (normally glucose or galactose).
d. **Further investigations**: generally only for bilateral cataract:
   1. Electrolytes (calcium, phosphorus)
   2. Amino acid titres

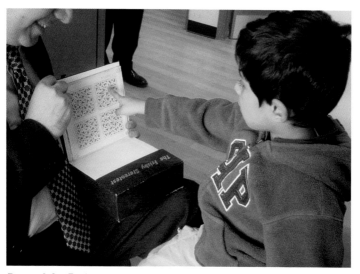

Figure 9.9 Frisby stereotest: good visual acuity and ocular alignment are essential to achieve good level of stereovision

3. Galactokinase levels
4. Other metabolic disease investigations.

E. Genetic and paediatric consultations

Dealing with bilateral cataract requires a multidisciplinary team, in which a paediatrician, geneticist and ophthalmologist work together to reach a systemic or syndromatic diagnosis. Chromosomal and genetic analysis may be required. Other specialists may need to be involved, including paediatric endocrinologists and dermatologists.

Parents frequently have questions about mortality, morbidity, inheritance and the chance of a second child with cataract. All these questions require a multidisciplinary team approach to be accurately answered.

Management

Management of paediatric cataract is a comprehensive process and starts from thorough assessment through to cataract surgery, followed by visual rehabilitation. It is frequently a challenge to maintain any immediate post-operative good visual outcome. The following sections outline the many key questions and points that should be addressed when considering the management of paediatric cataract.

Is it visually significant?

As mentioned earlier, not all congenital and infantile cataracts are visually significant. Therefore, careful assessment is vital in deciding those cases that need surgical intervention.

What is the prognosis?

Thorough examination can elicit signs that predict good visual outcomes, for example the absence of squint or nystagmus. However, slowly progressive cataracts (e.g. lamellar cataract, posterior lenticonus and PHPV) have better visual outcomes in comparison to congenital cataract that present as dense opacities from the start. That said, it can be notoriously difficult to predict the prognosis of a congenital cataract if left untreated. Nevertheless, tests such as serial red reflex photographs can help to decide the onset of visually significant cataract.

Not every congenital cataract requires surgery.

Signs of a favourable visual prognosis include:

- absence of strabismus or occular misalignment
- absence of nystagmus.

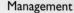
Surgical or conservative management?

It is important to classify whether a cataract is:

- not visually significant
- borderline, or
- visually significant.

There is no need to operate on a child that has a small or peripheral cataract in the presence of a good red reflex and good view of retinal blood vessels. If the cataract is minimally significant then dilating the pupil can often help to maintain good input to the visual pathway in the affected eye. Patching the good eye is important in this situation. Dilating eye drops can be either sympathomimetic agents, such as phenylephrine hydrochloride 2.5%, or parasympatholytic agents, such as tropicamide or atropine. The latter is usually given twice a week. The obvious risk of overtreatment with either penalization or patching is induced amblyopia. The majority of these cases end up with surgical removal of the cataract by age 2–3 years. If the cataract is visually significant then surgical intervention is obviously the best option. However, in all non-surgical cases, close follow is essential in order to detect early signs of amblyopia.

When to operate?

Visual deprivation due to congenital or infantile cataract can result in severe amblyopia that may be difficult to treat. Therefore, early intervention is essential whether this be for unilateral or bilateral cataract. Studies have shown high complication rates in children with congenital cataract who were operated at age 6 weeks or less. Conversely, delay in removing the cataract may result in severe amblyopia. Visually significant

---

- Overtreatment with patching or penalization therapy can result in deprivation or occlusion amblyopia in the sound eye.
- Frequent and close monitoring of children on amblyopia therapy is therefore essential.

paediatric cataract should be removed at age 4–6 weeks in unilateral cases and no later than 10 weeks in bilateral cases. In cases of bilateral cataract, only a small interval between the two cataract surgeries should be allowed in order to avoid the occurrence of amblyopia. The role of bilateral total patching for up to 2 weeks at a time, in neonates with bilateral congenital cataracts, based on its claim to prevent amblyopia remains controversial. Its use is reserved for cases where surgical intervention must be delayed, for example when a child's poor general health prevents safe anaesthesia.

Type of surgical intervention?

Techniques have evolved from intracapsular cataract extraction (known as lensectomy) to extracapsular cataract removal. This has the advantages of controlled anterior segment surgery and preservation of posterior capsule for primary or secondary lens implantation, and avoids vitreous loss. The lens material is usually soft and can be easily washed out through 'irrigation and aspiration' manoeuvres without the need for phacoemulsification (see Chapter 5).

Complications of paediatric cataract surgery

Children with cataract often have confounding anterior segment abnormalities. A combination of the inherent properties of an elastic eye in children and the presence of other abnormalities makes paediatric cataract surgery very challenging and a highly skilled procedure. The risk of complications due to the severe inflammatory response commonly encountered when performing surgeries on immature eyes is high. Such complications may be intra- or post-operative, some of the more common being as follows:

- **Intra-operative complications**: capsular tear, vitreous loss and choroidal haemorrhage.
- **Glaucoma**: the most commonly encountered type is pupil-block glaucoma, where the pupil is blocked either by vitreous or inflammatory membrane. Glaucoma can manifest many

years after the surgery. Ocular pain, watery eye, cloudy cornea (corneal oedema) and iris bombe are the signs that should be looked for on each visit, in particular at the first few post-operative visits. Intraocular pressure and the appearance of the optic discs should be checked. Refraction can show progressive myopic shift, which is another sign of progressive glaucoma. Aphakic glaucoma is more common than pseudophakic glaucoma in these patients.

- **Strabismus**: esotropia is more common in congenital cataracts, whereas exotropia is more common in acquired cataracts. Progressive strabismus after cataract surgery might indicate development of amblyopia.

- **Posterior capsule opacity**: the occurrence of posterior capsule opacity is 100% in children less than 1 year of age. Diminished red reflex, poor fixation and difficulty in refraction indicate the presence of posterior capsular opacity.

- **Amblyopia**: management of amblyopia is challenging. (It is discussed later in this chapter.)

- **Endophthalmitis**: can be devastating and the child can loose the eye.

- **Other post-operative complications**: wound leak, anterior synechiae, secondary uveitis, irregular pupil, dislocated intraocular lens (IOL), secondary inflammatory membranes, nystagmus, and posterior segment complications, such as vitreous haemorrhage and retinal detachment.

- Management of paediatric cataract surgery complications can be challenging. Post-operative medical intervention and further surgical procedures are often required.
- The most common post-operative complication is posterior capsular opacification, which can be dense and visually significant.
- Younger age and choice of surgical method play important roles in the development of posterior capsule opacity.
- Early detection and management of any post-operative visually significant opacification, such as posterior capsular opacity or presence of a fibrinous membrane, are essential for normal visual development.

Posterior capsule management

Posterior capsule opacification increases the risk of deprivation amblyopia. Furthermore, the younger the child, the more likely they are to develop clinically significant posterior capsule opacity. In fact, most children below 4 years of age will develop posterior capsular opacity that requires laser or surgical treatment. Primary posterior capsulorrhexis (surgical posterior capsulectomy) and anterior vitrectomy help to minimize the risk of posterior capsular opacity, which would obviously be difficult to treat by YAG-laser capsulotomy on an outpatient basis in the same way as for adults or for older children, where this can be easily carried out. Primary posterior capsulorrhexis and anterior vitrectomy is therefore performed in all children below 4 years of age.

Primary or secondary IOL implantation?

This remains a very controversial topic. Recent studies have shown favourable outcomes for primary IOL implantation (at the time of cataract removal). However, this can be technically difficult and very challenging in terms choosing the correct power of IOL and surgical positioning of the IOL. Secondary IOL implantation is safe and easier to perform in the fully grown eye. Acrylic, hydrophobic foldable IOLs are currently considered to be lens implants of choice. They have been shown to be superior in comparison with the traditionally used rigid polymethylmethacrylate (PMMA) IOLs when implanted in children's eyes. IOL power should be adjusted according to the age. For children less than 12–18 months of age, one should aim for hypermetropia of about 3–6 D. Above 2 years of age, it is generally recommended to aim for approximately 2 D of hyperopia.

Management of the aphakic child

Visual rehabilitation requires a clear visual axis and optical correction. Although advances in surgical techniques and types of IOLs have improved the outcomes of cataract surgery, optical correction following surgery, particularly for aphakic eyes, can be very challenging for the ophthalmologist, the optometrist and the family. Primary IOL implantation therefore minimizes the risk of severe debilitating amblyopia by reducing anisometropia. Aphakia may be corrected in children with contact lenses, spectacles, epikeratophakia or secondary IOL implantation. There are three main factors that decide the best methods of optical correction for the aphakic child: the age, the family and the status of the eye.

Contact lenses

Contact lenses remain the best option for children less than 2 years of age due to the difficulties associated with IOL implantation in neonates. They are used for bilateral, but more importantly unilateral, aphakia. They should be fitted as soon as possible after surgery (within a week if possible). The lens has to be changed frequently due to rapid growth of the eye within the first 2 years of life. Over-refraction is mandatory at each visit.

The following issues should be addressed when considering use of contact lenses for young children:

- **Power of lens**: it is important to ensure good near vision, especially in the first few years of age:
  - for children under 1 year of age add +3.00 D
  - for children between 1 and 2 years of age add +1 to +2 D
  - children over 2–3 years of age can be fitted with bifocals on top of their contact lenses (except in cases of unilateral aphakia).
- **Type of lens**
  - **Silicone contact lenses**: have very high oxygen permeability (high DK), which makes them suitable for long-term use because corneal hypoxemia may occur with the use of low oxygen permeability contact lenses. The disadvantages of these lenses, however, are their cost and their higher risk of contact-lens-related complications. Moreover, they are unable to correct high degrees of astigmatism. In addition, most parents find them difficult to use.

- **Silicone hydrogel contact lenses**: as the use of these materials increases, custom designs are now becoming available. They combine the benefits of silicone lenses with hydrogel material characteristics. Their use is widely anticipated to become the norm, particularly as the range of parameters available increases.
- **Rigid gas permeable (RGP) contact lenses**: have the advantage of correcting high degrees of astigmatism in addition to correcting aphakia. They are easy to use, but they are not easy to fit.
- **Hydrogel contact lenses**: are probably the most difficult to handle and their use is reserved mainly for neonates.
- **Compliance**: poor vision and uncooperative child can result in poor compliance. Parents should be continuously encouraged to persist with using contact lenses for their children.
- **Complications**: These have to be explained clearly to parents. Parents should be advised not to use the contact lenses if their child has red eye, irritation, discharge or any unusual findings in the cornea. Corneal hypoxemia (epithelial oedema and vascularization), infectious keratitis and corneal scarring are occasionally seen with long-term use of contact lens.

Spectacles

These are a good option for bilateral aphakia and are well tolerated by neonates as well as older children. They are considered a second choice to contact lenses, however, as an option in the management of unilateral aphakia.

- Visual rehabilitation is the next priority following removal of the visually significant cataract.
- Contact lenses can be as effective as intraocular lenses.
- Contact lens fitting and usage can be difficult for both practitioners and parents. It is important to give the parents all the support they need when handling contact lenses and dealing with complications.

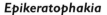
Epikeratophakia
Epikeratophakia is a type of onlay lamellar corneal graft that is hardly used nowadays. However, it remains an option in those who cannot tolerate contact lenses or spectacles and who are not suitable for secondary IOL implantation.

Secondary IOL implantation
Secondary IOL implantation is a great option, especially in cases of poor compliance or intolerance to contact lenses. (This option is discussed above.)

Amblyopia treatment

Treatment starts by creating a clear visual axis, which then should be followed by patching the dominating eye (occlusion therapy). The age of the child and the density of amblyopia both play a role in planning the most suitable patching regimen. Poor compliance of a child should not interfere with this decision.

The younger the child, the less patching is required. For a child up to 6 months of age, patching should not exceed 2 waking hours per day. However, some experts advise up to half the waking hours of the day. Bearing in mind that a newborn baby sleeps most of the day (waking hours are less than 4 hours on average), then total occlusion would not exceed the 2 hours already proposed.

With dense amblyopia, it is necessary to patch the good eye for longer hours.

Routine visual assessment, including observation of fixation behaviour, is important to monitor the response to treatment, detect early signs of occlusion amblyopia (amblyopia that

---

- The denser the amblyopia, the longer it is necessary to occlude the good eye.
- Visual behaviour is often the only way to assess the response to amblyopia therapy.
- Maintenance occlusion therapy may be necessary up to age 10 years of age.

develops in the occluded good eye) and adjust the occlusion regimen accordingly. Maintenance occlusion therapy may be necessary up to 9–10 years of age. If occlusion is not possible then an alternative treatment of penalizing the good eye may be considered. This consists of applying atropine twice a week to blur the image in the good eye. However, this is unlikely to be of benefit in cases of dense amblyopia, where the good eye will continue to have better vision despite penalization.

Family education and social circumstances

These factors have to be taken into consideration when planning paediatric cataract surgery. The need for surgery can be shocking news to the whole family. Support should be available throughout this period. The best way to deal with it is to educate the parents about:

- the possible causes of cataract in their child
- the need to operate at early age
- amblyopia risk and management
- surgical options
- postoperative care
- visual rehabilitation.

Conclusion

Paediatric cataract diagnosis and management differs from that of adult cataract. Early detection and treatment are the key factors for better visual outcomes. Delay in treatment might result in a legally registered blind child. There are two arms in the successful management of paediatric cataract:

- removal of the opacified lens, and
- appropriate visual rehabilitation.

It should always be borne in mind that congenital or childhood cataract can be the first presenting sign of a systemic disease.

Further reading

Amaya, L., Taylor, D., Russell-Eggitt, I., et al. (2003). The morphology and natural history of childhood cataracts. *Surv. Ophthalmol.* **48**: 125–144.

Cassidy, L., Rahi, J., Nischal, K., et al. (2001). Outcome of lens aspiration and intraocular lens implantation in children aged 5 years and under. *Br. J. Ophthalmol.* **85**: 540–542.

Drummond, G.T. and Hinz, B.J. (1994). Management of monocular cataract with long-term dilation in children. *Can. J. Ophthalmol.* **29**: 227–230.

Ellis, F.J. (2002). Management of pediatric cataract and lens opacities. *Curr. Opin. Ophthalmol.* **13**: 33–37.

Gimbel, H.V., Basti, S., Ferensowicz, M. and DeBroff, B.M. (1997). Results of bilateral cataract extraction with posterior chamber intraocular lens implantation in children. *Ophthalmology* **104**: 1737–1743.

Hamill, M.B. and Koch, D.D. (1999). Pediatric cataracts. *Curr. Opin. Ophthalmol.* **10**: 4–9.

Hiles, D.A. (1984). Intraocular lens implantation in children with monocular cataracts. *Ophthalmology* **91**: 1231–1238.

Jain, I.S., Pillai, P., Gangwar, D.N., et al. (1983). Congenital cataract; etiology and morphology. *J. Pediatr. Ophthalmol. Strabismus* **20**: 238–242.

Jensen, A.A., Basti, S., Greenwald, M.J. and Mets, M.B. (2002). When may the posterior capsule be preserved in pediatric intraocular lens surgery? *Ophthalmology* **109**: 324–327.

Kuchle, M., Lausen, B. and Gusek–Schneider, G.C. (2003). Results and complications of hydrophobic acrylic vs PMMA posterior chamber lenses in children under 17 years of age. *Graefe's Arch. Clin. Exp. Ophthalmol.* **241**: 637–641.

Lundvall, A. and Zetterstrom, C. (1999). Complications after early surgery for congenital cataracts. *Acta Ophthalmol. Scand.* **77**: 677–680.

Marner, E., Rosenberg, T. and Eiberg, H. (1989). Autosomal dominant congenital cataract. morphology and genetic mapping. *Acta Ophthalmol.* **67**: 151–158.

Moore, B.D. (1989). Changes in the aphakic refraction of children with unilateral congenital cataracts. *J. Pediatr. Ophthalmol. Strabismus* **26**: 290–295.

Moore, B.D. (1993). Pediatric aphakic contact lens wear: rates of successful wear. *J. Pediatr. Ophthalmol. Strabismus* **30**: 253–258.

Moore, B.D. (1994). Optometric management of congenital cataracts. *J. Am. Optom. Assoc.* **65**: 719–724.

Moore, B.D. (1994). Pediatric cataracts – diagnosis and treatment. *Optom. Vis. Sci.* **71**:168–173.

Morgan, K.S. (1995). Pediatric cataract and lens implantation. *Curr. Opin. Ophthalmol.* **6**: 9–13.

Neumann, D., Weissman, B.A., Isenberg, S.J., et al. (1993). The effectiveness of daily wear contact lenses for the correction of infantile aphakia. *Arch. Ophthalmol.* **111**: 927–930.

O'Keefe, M., Fenton, S. and Lanigan, B. (2001). Visual outcomes and complications of posterior chamber intraocular lens implantation in the first year of life. *J. Cataract Refract. Surg.* **27**: 2006–2011.

Rowe, N.A., Biswas, S. and Lloyd, I.C. (2004). Primary IOL implantation in children: a risk analysis of foldable acrylic v PMMA lenses. *Br. J. Ophthalmol.* **88**: 481–485.

Taylor, D.S.I. (1997). *Paediatric Ophthalmology*, 2nd edition. Blackwell Science, pp. 461–476.

Taylor, D., Wright, K.W., Amaya, L., et al. (2001). Should we aggressively treat unilateral congenital cataracts? *Br. J. Ophthalmol.* **85**: 1120–1126.

Wang, V.M., Demer, J.L., Rosenbaum, A. and Weissman, B.A. (2002). Diagnosing glaucoma in pediatric aphakia. *Optometry* **73**: 704–710.

Wilson, M.E., Jr., Bartholomew, L.R. and Trivedi, R.H. (2003). Pediatric cataract surgery and intraocular lens implantation: practice styles and preferences of the 2001 ASCRS and AAPOS memberships. *J. Cataract. Refract. Surg.* **29**: 1811–1820.

Wright, K. (2002). Lens abnormalities. In: *Pediatric Ophthalmology and Strabismus*, 2nd edition. Ed: Wright, K.W., Spiegel, P.H. Springer-Verlag, Chapter 27.

Wright, K.W. (1997). Pediatric cataracts. *Curr. Opin. Ophthalmol.* **8**: 50–55.

Wright, K.W., Edelman, P.M., Walonker, F. and Yiu, S. (1986). Reliability of fixation preference testing in diagnosing amblyopia. *Arch. Ophthalmol.* **104**: 549–553.

Wright, K.W., Walonker, F. and Edelman, P. (1981). 10-Diopter fixation test for amblyopia. *Arch. Ophthalmol.* **99**: 1242–1246.

10

The future of cataract surgery management

Richard Packard and Helen Pointer

Introduction

In 1970, when one of the authors began their career in ophthalmology, cataract surgery and patient management were very different from today. The cataract was removed intact through a 180-degree incision and two or three silk sutures were inserted to close the eye. The surgery was carried out without gloves, often with no magnifying aids and, with a very few exceptions, no intraocular lens was inserted. Patients were normally nursed in bed and only discharged 7–10 days after the operation. They had strict instructions as to what they could and could not do. Although contact lenses existed they were large haptic ones and few patients were prepared to use them. This meant that patients required aphakic spectacles usually in powers around +12°D. They were thus effectively ocular cripples as these glasses influenced their lifestyle considerably. As a result most patients were not operated upon until both cataracts were well advanced and could both be removed. Demand was limited, but despite this there were waiting lists due to the relatively small number of surgeons.

How things have changed today. As a result of the work of Charles Kelman in the late 1960s to develop phacoemulsification, and after the early work of Harold Ridley in the 1950s to advance the design and materials of intraocular lenses, surgery is dramatically different. Incisions have got smaller and smaller so that most cataract operations are performed through incisions less than 3 mm, with minimally invasive anaesthesia using topical gel or drops. The surgery itself is much safer and with very few complications due to improvements in technology. Further, with advances in phacoemulsification power delivery, it is possible to do this using incisions of less than 1.5 mm. Foldable intraocular lenses can be inserted through 2 mm or even smaller incisions with good visual results and multifocal lenses are being used in greater numbers.

These advances in cataract surgery have led to unprecedented demand as patients have realized what can be done for them. Surgery is carried out much earlier than previously, with symptomatic patients with 6/9 or sometimes better vision being found on most operating lists. Very few patients now stay in hospital for longer than a few hours and follow-up visits are being reduced further and further.

All of these changes have led to a variety of differing approaches to patient management. It is anticipated there will be a number of different models for the pathway a patient will follow between symptoms of cataract being perceived by the patient and referral for surgery and post-operative follow up. This chapter explores some of these options and shows how the role of the optometrist may change to become an important part of the whole.

Traditional model

The system that had applied generally until the past few years (and still applies in many areas) was that when a patient was advised they had a cataract by their primary care practitioner, be that general practitioner (GP), optometrist or ophthalmic medical practitioner, they would be referred for an outpatient appointment at the nearest eye department. The pathway would be as follows:

1. Having already been advised of the presence of cataract the patient would be seen at the eye department and be told they had cataract. A little frustrating perhaps since confirmation of the diagnosis would be all they achieved at this appointment. If appropriate, there would then be a discussion about surgery:
   - if the patient consented at this appointment they would then be added to the waiting list; the approximate wait would have been 12–18 months, although it is now down to 3 months.
   - if the patient decided not to go ahead with surgery they possibly would be reviewed by the eye department until such time as this changed, or most likely they would be returned to the community for monitoring.

Primary care practitioners, aware of the lengthy waiting times, would often refer a little early so that their patient could get in the queue and would be ready for surgery by the time their name came up. However this would not always work because if the patient was called too early they would not be offered surgery.

2. Closer to the time of surgery, the patient would have to attend the eye department for biometry and formal consent. They would then have surgery, usually as a daycase procedure.

3. Within 48 hours of surgery the patient would be contacted, and in some areas they would be seen by the eye department for a post-operative assessment. At 2 weeks after surgery the patient would have a clinic appointment for a post-surgical examination.

4. At 5–6 weeks the patient would be asked to visit their optician for refraction and new glasses.

Although this type of approach is still in use in a number of areas, things are rapidly changing, both in the pathway from diagnosis to follow-up and in terms of who does what to whom and where. Several Department of Health initiatives, and also changes in the legislation governing the way in which optometrists can practise, have opened up the possibilities, enabling this and other pathways to take off. Not only are the referral pathways changing but also the types of facility and surgical personnel involved and will alter further.

Direct optometric referral and shared care post-operatively

For some years optometrists have been able to decide whether a patient needs to be referred to a medical practitioner. Prior to this time General Optical Council regulations stipulated that an optometrist must refer when an abnormality is detected. In addition, the regulations altered again in 2005 such that optometrists are now permitted to refer for any condition directly to an eye department, with a copy of that referral going to the patient's GP. Previously the only route for referral to an dye department was via the GP.

The patient's pathway under the new arrangements is as follows:

1. The patient is monitored closely in the community until such time as the patient feels surgery is necessary. The decision to refer is made after discussion about the risks involved, and since the patient will have to be offered a choice of where to have their cataract surgery the referral is often directed through a referral management centre. The most important aspect of the direct referral is the appropriateness of that referral, the criteria being:
   - the patient has a cataract
   - the cataract is affecting the patient's quality of life
   - you have discussed the risks and benefits of cataract surgery with the patient, and
   - the patient would like to have cataract surgery.
2. Once the eye department has been chosen the patient can then visit for one pre-operative biometry appointment, at which consent for surgery is agreed with the consultant. The cataract assessment clinics prepare patients for cataract surgery. If the patient does not want an operation then the appointment is unnecessary. In this event, the patient should be asked to return to their optometrist once everyday aspects of their lives have become affected by their poor vision and they are prepared to accept the risks and benefits of cataract extraction.
3. The next and only other visit to the eye department will then be for the operation.
4. After surgery the patient is contacted to ensure all is well at 24–48 hours and the next practitioner to examine them is their community optometrist at 4–6 weeks. This appointment is combined with a post-operative refraction.

Training requirements for optometric direct referral

For optometrists to become involved in the referral pathway there will need to be some training, however this will not need to be extensive. The most important requirement for direct referral is a better understanding of when a patient is likely to be turned down for surgery. Until recently optometrists were compelled to refer any and all stages of cataracts under regulations, but now the expectation is that they hold on to patients with even quite advanced cataracts until it is appropriate for the patient to have surgery. This change in culture for optometrists presents the greatest difference in mindset.

While optometrists have no difficulty in detecting cataract it becomes increasingly important to dilate the pupil as the cataract develops. Without this, a thorough fundus examination cannot be performed and those with both age-related macular degeneration and cataracts, for example, may be given a falsely optimistic expectation of their vision after surgery. Funding for this extended examination is not available in all areas. However in those areas that do fund this service the accuracy of optometric referrals is very high.

Training packages for optometrists vary around the country, but in general they involve sessions in the eye department, watching and taking part in pre-operative and post-operative clinics and also watching at least one session in theatre. The session in theatre is mainly so that those involved are able to describe the set-up adequately to their patients. The pre-operative session is helpful, as having heard the consultant obtain consent for surgery from a patient the optometrist will then be able to use a similar form of words when they need to get a patient's permission to refer. Furthermore, if the optometrist describes the risks adequately, in the same way as the consultant would have later on, the patient may decide against surgery at that pre-operative session, so avoiding wasting the patient's time at an outpatient appointment.

Post-operative care is really where optometrists are taking on more responsibility than in the past. This role has already been delegated to ophthalmic nurses in many areas, but removing it one stage further, to the community optometrist, is a new development. Optometrists usually only see patients at 6 weeks, but at 4 weeks an eye may look different. A post-operative session in the eye department plus a lecture including slides is generally used to ensure competency for this part of the pathway.

Appendices 10.1 to 10.6 give an example of a current shared-care scheme for direct optometry referral and post-operative follow-up used by The Queen Victoria Hospital, East Grinstead, and Sussex Eye Hospital, Brighton.

Models of cataract surgical delivery

As has been shown, cataract pathways are altering to involve the optometrist more in pre- and post-operative roles. At the same time, the Department of Health has been introducing the idea of patient choice. Thus at the point of entry into the system, whether this be in the GP's surgery or the optometrist's premises, the patient will be offered choices as to the providers of their cataract assessment and surgery. It is envisaged that a software system called 'Choose and Book' will facilitate this process. Five choices will be available, of which one should be a private sector provider. It is envisaged that in practice most patients will choose their local NHS hospital, now that waiting times have come down considerably. However if a provider cannot meet its targets for waiting times, possibly because it has become too busy for its capacity or is inefficient, its names will not be available as a choice until its waiting times are back on target. Another programme, called 'Payment by Results', is also being introduced. Each procedure or service will have a tariff price, and thus surgical facilities will only get paid for the number of procedures carried out. As stated, a variety of providers is envisaged for cataract surgery:

- traditional full-service NHS hospital eye departments
- NHS treatment centres
- independent treatment centres (ISTC)
- private hospitals, both bidding for NHS contract work and continuing to do traditional private surgery.

In this scenario, NHS hospitals may be at a disadvantage in terms of throughput per operating list as they will need to continue to train surgeons for the next generation. Although the Government is considering asking ISTCs, etc., to provide surgical training, in practice this will be unpopular where a commercial organization is concerned. Two main models of purchasing are being considered. Primary care trusts have, until now, been using block contracts to commission work, but this will change as Choose and Book is rolled out. Practice-based commissioning will be introduced to allow individual GP practices to purchase directly from providers, who will be reimbursed under Payment by Results.

It remains to be seen how well these various changes will work in practice. There are certainly more initiatives being explored in other parts of ophthalmology, for example 'Do Once and Share' (DOAS), which will involve community optometrists in direct patient care. The DOAS programme (www.rcophth.ac.uk/about/college/doas-cataract) seeks to avoid unnecessary duplication of effort by enabling clinicians to share their experience once at a national level and to contribute, with colleagues, to best practice and a national approach to ophthalmic care for patients with cataracts.

National consultations have been undertaken in order to create the best practice model, and this new approach to care will aim to make optimum use of new information technology systems to allow information recorded by GPs, optometrists and ophthalmologists to be shared. This will help to improve current practice by providing benchmark standards and reduce inconsistencies nationwide for optometrists, the majority of whom may eventually be involved in the DOAS cataract care pathway.

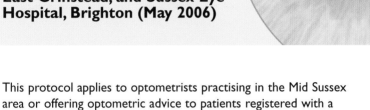

Appendix 10.1

An example of a current shared-care scheme for direct optometry referral and post-operative follow-up used by The Queen Victoria Hospital, East Grinstead, and Sussex Eye Hospital, Brighton (May 2006)

This protocol applies to optometrists practising in the Mid Sussex area or offering optometric advice to patients registered with a general practitioner (GP) in Mid Sussex. Neighbouring primary care trusts (PCTs) have similar schemes.

Optometrists are asked to refer patients direct to hospitals via the PCT's Primary Care Commissioning Centre (PCCC). A Patient Care Adviser (PCA) at PCCC will then discuss choice with the patient and send the referral on to the hospital of choice. The PCA will also send a copy of the referral to the patient's GP. The optometrist receives a fee for direct referral. Accredited optometrists, whose patient subsequently attends either the Sussex Eye Hospital, Brighton, or The Queen Victoria Hospital, East Grinstead, for surgery can also claim a fee for undertaking the patient follow-up at 4–6 weeks post surgery. The fees will be authorized by the PCT and passed to the Primary Care Support Centre, based in Worthing, for payment. This is the same team that processes NHS sight tests and vouchers.

The options for surgery for Mid Sussex patients are currently Queen Victoria Hospital, East Grinstead, and Sussex Eye Hospital, Brighton. Practices are provided with two leaflets to give to patients who are referred. The first is an RNIB leaflet to help the patients understand what a cataract is. The second leaflet is about choice and the local providers.

Optometrists and ophthalmic medical practitioners (OMPs) who wish to be involved in the scheme are required to register their interest in using the pathway for direct referral by signing the PCT Service Level Agreement (Appendix 10.2). They must then go through the following accreditation process before they start providing post-operative assessment.

To register their desire to train to become an accredited practitioner the PCT coordinator, who will record the practitioner's name, practice and GOC number, or in the case of an OMP their GMC number and contact details. The practitioner will then be sent an accreditation card to take to the hospital to record training undertaken.

For accreditation training, each practitioner must:

- watch a pre-operative clinic session
- watch at least three cataract operations
- observe one post-operative patient soon after cataract surgery
- attend a post-operative session
- attend accreditation lectures, and
- undertake an accreditation assessment (Appendix 10.3).

OMPs are not required to watch clinics or surgery but may do so if they wish.

The accreditation card issued to a training practitioner by the PCT has to be signed by the person taking the clinic or theatre once the training has been completed. Photographic proof of identity is required. Once completed the card is returned to the PCT coordinator. Eleven DOCET (Directorate of Optometric Continuing Education and Training) points are awarded for the whole accreditation process.

A discussion with the optometrist or OMP prior to surgery about the desired spectacle refraction after surgery and the potential for post-operative anisometropia between the first eye and second eye should be had before referral. The final planned prescription is almost always plano to −1.0 D, so if this will be a problem between eyes some of the ways of solving this, for example contact lenses, should be explained, even if it will only be a short-term problem.

Optometrists are advised to complete a referral form (Appendix 10.4) only if the patient has decided that they wish to have surgery. The optometrist should complete the referral form and fax it to the PCA on the number on the form. The GP's name and address is required on the form so that the PCA can send a copy of the referral on to the patient's GP. The optometrist is also expected to provide the patient with leaflets from the RNIB about cataracts and also to request that the patient bring an up-to-date list of medication to the hospital at their pre-operative visit (Appendix 10.5).

Bearing in mind that the dates for pre-operative assessment and surgery may be 3–4 months from the date of referral, the optometrist is requested to state any unsuitable dates for the patient. For example, if the patient is away all winter or will be away at around that time.

As the patient's primary eye care practitioner, often their optometrist or OMP is more aware of their likely preferred refraction following surgery. There is also often more chance to discuss this before referral, and therefore if there is a desired refraction then this needs to be stated in the comments box.

If the referral is for a second eye, the optometrist is advised to mark this clearly in the comments box so that the patient's previous notes are found and a new set not made. Often the biometry readings will already have been taken.

On receipt of referral, the PCA faxes a copy to the patient's GP requesting completion of the medical issues box within 72 hours. Within 3 days of receipt the PCA will contact the patient to discuss their choice and notify current waiting times.

The referral is posted first class to the chosen provider and the optometrist is notified by fax as to which provider has been chosen. In order to maintain patient confidentiality, the fax will only contain the patient's initials.

On a quarterly basis the number of referrals per practice is collated to trigger the initial referral fee payment, which is paid by the Primary Care Support Centre.

Surgery takes place after one pre-operative clinic, and unless there are any complications the patient is referred back for a post-operative appointment and post-operative refraction with the referring optometrist or OMP (for which the usual General Ophthalmic Services (GOS) ST fee may be claimed) where the referring practitioner is accredited for post-operative shared care with the hospital. The patient attends with a post-operative form (Appendix 10.6), which would also have been faxed from the hospital. This must be completed and returned to the hospital. The final part of this form is the trigger for the practitioner to be paid for performing the post-operative appointment.

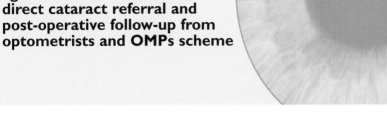

Appendix 10.2

Example of a service level agreement for a combined direct cataract referral and post-operative follow-up from optometrists and OMPs scheme

Optometrists/OMPs wishing to participate in the scheme must undertake an appropriate accreditation programme and agree to work to the following protocol when assessing, referring and following up patients.

An initial assessment of the patient must be carried out. This would normally include a routine sight test. If the optometrist/OMP considers that the patient will benefit from cataract surgery (visual acuity worse than 6/9, except in exceptional circumstances), the following protocol must be used:

1. Discuss with the patient whether the cataract is affecting their quality of life.
2. Assess any ocular co-morbidity and risk factors for a poor outcome following cataract surgery, including systemic medication.
3. Explain the basic process of phacoemulsification cataract surgery and the general risks and benefits.
4. Establish that the patient wants to have cataract surgery within the next few months.
5. Give the patient the information leaflets *Understanding Cataracts* and *Mid Sussex PCT Cataract Provider Information*, and explain to them that this tells them how to book their appointment.

Where the optometrist/OMP does not consider that the patient will significantly benefit from surgery, or the patient is unwilling to undergo the procedure at present, the patient should continue to be managed in the normal way.

This scheme is only designed for those patients whose principal problem is cataract. All other referrals should be dealt with in the normal way.

Should the patient wish to be referred to a hospital outside the scheme, then the patient should be referred to their GP and the referral will be made by the GP.

This service is only applicable to patients who live within the Mid Sussex PCT area.

Following the assessment, fill in the Referral Form for Cataract Surgery. All relevant information, patient details and current Rx must be fully completed.

- Part I: fax or post a copy to the Primary Care Commissioning Centre and then keep for your own records.
- Part II: send to the patient's GP.

This service will be subject to clinical governance and the normal Post Payment Verification process.

Follow-up procedure

A Community Post Cataract Operation Report Form will be sent to you, following your patient's operation. The patient will be told to contact you for an appointment at four weeks. If the patient has not made contact by the fifth week you will need to contact them to book an appointment. If they have not attended for their follow-up appointment by the end of the eighth week please report back to the Cataract Coordinator.

Once you have seen the patient you should complete and return the form to the Cataract Coordinator at the relevant hospital.

Where the patient presents with a post-operative problem that requires an ophthalmologist's opinion, contact the relevant hospital to ensure that the patient is referred back in as appropriate.

The Agreement

- I agree to work to this protocol when assessing, referring and following up patients for the Mid Sussex Cataract Choice Referral Service.

Signature of senior clinician:

Name:

GOC/GMC number:

Date:

SPECIALIST PROJECT CONFIDENTIALITY NOTICE

ASSIGNMENT: MID SUSSEX PCT REFERRAL MANAGEMENT

LOCATION: MID SUSSEX PCT HQ

During your assignment you may gain privileged knowledge of a highly confidential nature relating to the private affairs, diagnosis and treatment of patients, information affecting members of the public, general practitioners and items under consideration by the PCT.

You are not permitted to disclose such information outside the PCT's procedures.

Breaches of confidence or other failures to comply with the PCT's procedures and the Data Protection Act 1998 will result in the immediate termination of your assignment, possible disciplinary action and may also lead to legal proceedings.

Agreement

I agree to adhere to the PCT's policies in relation to Data Protection and Information Security. I will not disclose any privileged, sensitive or confidential information to any unauthorized person. I understand the conditions and principles of processing personal data in relation to the Data Protection Act 1998. I understand and agree to abide by the requirements around confidentiality.

Signed:

Date:

Appendix 10.3
Example of questions asked for an accreditation assessment in order to ensure a minimum standard of knowledge

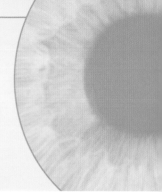

1. Which of the following does NOT increase the risk of post-operative corneal oedema after cataract surgery?
   a. pre-existing endothelial dystrophy
   b. intraoperative endothelial trauma
   c. raised intraocular pressure
   d. amblyopia
   e. endophthalmitis

2. A patient presents with an intraocular pressure of 4 mmHg after cataract surgery. Typical potential findings do NOT include:
   a. iris prolapse
   b. flat anterior chamber
   c. tense proptosis
   d. retinal detachment
   e. choroidal effusion

3. At the 6-week post-operative check following routine phacoemulsification cataract surgery, which of the following findings do NOT require referral back to the eye department?
   a. subconjunctival haemorrhage
   b. intraocular pressure (IOP) of 30 mmHg or greater
   c. Seidel positive test
   d. corneal sutures still present
   e. anterior chamber activity present (>2 cells seen in a 2 × 2 mm field)
   f. residual diplopia during up gaze only

4. Which of the two following systemic medications may predispose to complications during cataract surgery and therefore require alteration in dose or regime prior to surgery?
   a. tamsulosin (Flomax)
   b. warfarin
   c. aspirin
   d. analgesia
   e. cholesterol-lowering medication

5. In the majority of cases, phacoemulsification cataract surgery is usually performed under which of the two following techniques?
   a. general anaesthesia
   b. peribulbar local anaesthesia
   c. topical anaesthesia
   d. sub-Tenon's local anaesthesia

6. Which of the parameters below are essential in order to calculate the required power of an intraocular lens implant?
   a. keratometry
   b. axial length
   c. pre-operative refraction in the eye requiring surgery
   d. pupil diameter
   e. pachymetry

7. Which of the following (a–f) is correct?
   Within 24 hours following cataract surgery, the patient may experience:
   a. a dull ache or discomfort
   b. 'pins and needles' and tiredness, if acetazolamide has been prescribed
   c. slight blurred vision
   d. diplopia
   e. all of the above
   f. none of the above

8. Progression of age-related macular degeneration from 'dry' to 'wet' with choroidal neovascular membrane is a recognized complication of routine phacoemulsification cataract surgery. True or False?

9. Progression of diabetic retinopathy is a recognized complication of routine phacoemulsification cataract surgery. True or False?

10. At the 6-week post-operative check following routine phacoemulsification cataract surgery, if corrected visual acuity is 6/12 or better then it is not essential to perform a dilated retinal examination, even in patients known to have background diabetic retinopathy or dry age-related macular degeneration. True or False?

Appendix 10.4
Example of a direct referral form

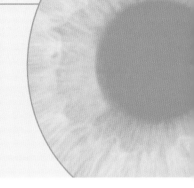

*Please print clearly in capitals – form for faxing

PATIENT DETAILS

Surname:	First name:	Title:
Address:	D.O.B.	Sex: ☐ M ☐ F
	NHS no:	
	Day time tel. no:	
	Best time to call patient:	
Postcode:	Other information (e.g. communication needs, carer details):	

GP DETAILS   **PCCC use only**

GP Name:	PCT:
Address:	Tel. No:
	Fax. No:

TO BE COMPLETED BY THE OPTOMETRIST/OMP
Please complete *all* information *clearly* to receive payment

☐ This patient has a cataract
☐ The cataract is causing the patient visual symptoms such that the quality of life is impaired e.g. for driving, reading, sewing, etc.
☐ I have explained the cataract surgery process, the *risks/benefits* and given the booklets
☐ The patient wishes to undergo cataract surgery under local anaesthetic
☐ The patient will need a general anaesthetic and/or is unsuitable for day surgery**
   **see back of form for criteria

Please indicate the patient's need for surgery in which eye:
☐ left eye   ☐ right eye   ☐ both eyes, priority being: ☐ left   ☐ right

Refraction details from current sight test

	V	Sph	Cyl	Axis	Prism	Base	VA	Add	Near VA
RE									
LE									

Other ocular pathology, i.e. amblyopia and relevant information:

Examination findings:

Anterior segment:

IOP (and instrument used):

Dilated fundus examination:

Comments (please include current medication – including eye drops, etc. – allergies or relevant medical or social issues):

OPTOMETRIST/OMP DETAILS

Name:	Optometrist/OMP-GOC/GMC No:
Address:	Accredited: ☐ Brighton ☐ Worthing ☐ East Grinstead ☐ Other – please state below.

I declare that the information I have given on this form is correct and complete and I understand that if it is not, action may be taken against me. For the purpose of verification of this claim, I consent to the disclosure of relevant information. I claim payment of fees due to me for work carried out under this NHS scheme.

Signature:

Date:

Print:

Appendix 10.5
Example of a patient letter at the time of referral to the hospital

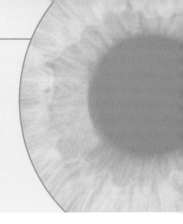

To be printed on optician's own headed paper or at least to be typed with their contact details in this top corner.

date

Dear *Patient's name*,

I have today referred you for cataract surgery. You may now choose where you have your cataract surgery, and very shortly you will be contacted by our patient advisers who will discuss your choices with you. I have given you a booklet about your options.

If at any time in the next few weeks you have doubts about going ahead with the surgery, please contact me so we can discuss your concerns. If you have second thoughts I can arrange for you to be taken off the list for surgery and we will continue to monitor your cataract development here.

Please remember to take a list of your current medication with you to your first appointment. (Your GP surgery can print this off for you if you do not have an up to date list.) Your operation will take place very soon after the initial appointment for measurements and you will be directed back to me for a health check up and new glasses prescription.

I am enclosing a leaflet from the RNIB about cataracts that contains some helpful information.

Yours sincerely,

Name of optometrist

Appendix 10.6
An example a community post-cataract operation report form

PATIENT DETAILS (please print)

Surname:	First name:	
Address:	D.O.B.	
	Male	Female
	Tel. nos:	
	NHS number:	
Postcode:	Date of visit:	

The above named patient underwent RIGHT/LEFT cataract surgery on   /   /

Routine: Yes   If No, explain

Lens implant used and power:

Refraction aimed for:

The surgery was carried out at:
• Queen Victoria Hospital, East Grinstead   ☐
• Sussex Eye Hospital, Brighton   ☐

Please complete the following and return to the appropriate hospital.

	RIGHT	**LEFT**
Unaided visions	6/	6/
REFRACTION		
(plus cyl form) SPH		
Cyl and axis		
Best corrected VA	6/	6/
Near ADD		
Near VA		
SLIT-LAMP EXAM		
Eyelids		
Conjunctiva		
Cornea		
Anterior chamber		
Pupil		
IOL		
Tonometry reading		
Instrument used		
Dilated fundus		
Examination		
Drops used		
Lens used		

Anterior segment findings

Additional comments:

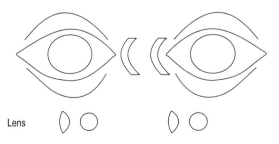

Lens

Dilated fundus examination

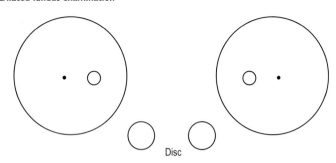

Disc

Quality standards

Has or does the patient give a history of pain, discomfort or sudden reduction in vision?

Wound red or unusual in any way?

Intolerable or unacceptable astigmatism?

Intolerable or unacceptable anisometropia?

Corrected acuity <post-op PH or <6/12?

IOP (mmHg) Goldmann/NCT/Perkins R _____ mmHg L _____ mmHg

Slit lamp

Anterior chamber activity present? (>2 cells seen in 2 × 2 mm field)

Cornea not clear?

Posterior synechiae?

Thickening of posterior capsule?

Any vitreous activity?

Are any sutures protruding or loose?

Examination not carried out (reason):

Index

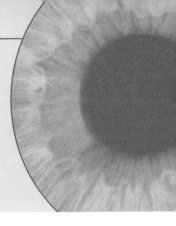